promoting healthy behaviour

promoting
healthy
behaviour

a practical guide for nursing and healthcare professionals

Professor Dominic Upton
Head of Psychological Sciences,
University of Worcester

Dr Katie Thirlaway
Head of the Department of Psychology,
University of Wales Institute, Cardiff

Harlow, England • London • New York • Boston • San Francisco • Toronto • Sydney • Singapore • Hong Kong
Tokyo • Seoul • Taipei • New Delhi • Cape Town • Madrid • Mexico City • Amsterdam • Munich • Paris • Milan

Pearson Education Limited
Edinburgh Gate
Harlow
Essex CM20 2JE
England

and Associated Companies throughout the world

Visit us on the World Wide Web at:
www.pearsoned.co.uk

First published 2010

ISBN: 978-0-273-72385-1

British Library Cataloguing-in-Publication Data
A catalogue record for this book is available from the British Library

Library of Congress Cataloging-in-Publication Data
Upton, Dominic.
   Promoting healthy behaviour : a practical guide for nursing and healthcare / Dominic Upton,
Katie Thirlaway.
       p. ; cm.
   Includes bibliographical references and index.
   ISBN 978-0-273-72385-1 (pbk.)
   1. Health promotion. 2. Nursing. I. Thirlaway, Kathryn. II. Title.
   [DNLM: 1. Health Behavior. 2. Health Promotion—methods. 3. Life Style. 4. Nurse's
Role. W 85 U71p 2010]
   RA427.8.U68 2010
   613—dc22

                                                                          2010004226

10 9 8 7 6 5 4 3 2 1
14 13 12 11 10

Typeset in 9pt and Interstate-Light font by 75
Printed in Great Britain by Henry Ling Ltd., at the Dorset Press, Dorchester, Dorset

For Penney (DU)

For Mark (KT)

Contents

Preface

Background to this book

In 2009 we published a well-received text on *The Psychology of Lifestyle* (Thirlaway and Upton, 2009) which was based on our experience and understanding of the major challenges that faced the UK – and the wider Western world – in terms of the so-called 'lifestyle diseases'. During the writing of that text we both became convinced that there was a need for a book that had a practical focus, albeit within an academic and evidence base framework: the result was this text.

The rationale for this book (and the previous one) was based on the premise that 'lifestyle diseases' are one of the major challenges facing the NHS. This is not a supposition put forward by ourselves exclusively but by many others, including not least the former prime minister, Tony Blair. Of course, politicians are not the only ones to have entered the debate. Opinion formers, academics and leader writers have all contributed to the debate, with increasing attention given to these diseases, whether this be within academia, social policy or the media. We and many others have long recognised the importance of psychology in the development of these lifestyle diseases and we wanted to ensure that appropriate psychological theory and practice were discussed and disseminated for use as part of the armoury available for healthcare professionals. Further research and discussion with colleagues led us to believe that there was a market for such a book and we began a dialogue with a very receptive publisher from which this text has resulted.

It has been appreciated for some time that poor lifestyles are associated with increasing health risk – at both an individual and a population level. Of course, such diseases are not distributed evenly across the population; there are certain sections of society that may suffer more than others. Hence, the influence of social class, gender and ethnicity should not be overlooked. It is essential that all healthcare professionals take into account these variables when discussing some of the approaches in this text. Furthermore, it is obvious that cognisance has to be taken of the individual differences when in a clinical situation; the personal characteristics and situation of the individual client can have a significant bearing on an individual's health and lifestyle. These characteristics may be related to their current situation or may be related to more cultural aspects. Moreover, there are differences between the individual countries of the UK, with certain behaviours and health and illnesses more prominent in some areas compared to others. There are also psychological variables which may be described as either 'risk' factors or 'protective' factors – 'personality' variables, self-efficacy or mood, for example.

Psychological models have attempted to integrate all of these social, demographic and psychological variables to predict behaviours and develop theoretically based interventions. This has been the fundamental foundation of this text. We have tried to demonstrate the value of these psychological models and how they can be used practically by healthcare professionals.

We see the role of psychology in lifestyle as of significant, if not of primary, importance. Similarly, we see the role of lifestyle in health and in illness as predominating and likely to become ever more important to the NHS in the coming decades. Indeed, the Foresight report described the 'obesity epidemic' as a problem comparable to climate change (Jones *et al.*, 2007). Obviously, how these issues are going to be addressed is a matter of debate and potential solutions range from the theoretically driven to the more light-hearted. Lifestyle is an issue about which every commentator feels confident to express an opinion. For example, the stigmatisation of obese people (albeit in, one would assume, a humorous article) is not uncommon: 'Most obesity is a consequence of stupidity and indolence and not of some genetic affliction. It is a lifestyle choice which people would be less inclined to adopt if they knew we all hated them for it' (Liddle, 2008). In this text, we review some of the more serious and theoretically driven approaches, debate their value and discuss the potential ways that healthcare professionals can use these for the benefit of their patients and clients.

Overall, we hope that you find this book useful and informative and a guide for your practice both now and in the future. It is geared towards healthcare professionals at any stage of their careers: those wishing to enter a health education/promotion, health (or social) care profession, those new to their particular role and those who have been engaged in professional practice for a number of years but wish to enhance their practice. It is not a manual of tips or a series of laws that have to be followed by all. There are some methods and guiding principles that we hope you will find useful, but this text is intended to be a series of thought-provoking chapters that will intrigue, stimulate and provoke, and hopefully enhance your practice for the benefit of your patients and clients.

The content of this book

We thought for some time about the content of this book – what should we include and what should be excluded? We also had advice from others who suggested additional material, but then others suggested other forms of behaviour that could be included. For example, should we include sleeping? After all, it is a behaviour and can affect health either positively or negatively. Similarly, others considered that we should include stress, which can impact on both mental and physical health and contributes significant mortality through accidents.

We also knew the psychology that needed to be included. So what was the cause of our consternation? Why did we spend so much time discussing the content over well-brewed coffee (other than the obvious)? We appreciated at the outset that there was a possibility of considerable repetition within this text. Many of the behaviours discussed are underpinned by similar psychological variables and have been investigated within similar theoretical modes. After writing the first couple of chapters we recognised this and re-jigged the book to include the chapter on psychological concepts, which presents the information in a more coherent and sensible manner. We hope that this has removed considerable overlap, although we recognise that there are key psychological principles and models which will play a central part in many of the behaviours we discuss.

We should emphasise at the outset that this is not a book about smoking or obesity or psychological concepts *alone*. It is a book that attempts to cover a range of topics in an integrating framework. Hence, there are sections on social support, for example, that some may consider skimpy, and there are psychological factors and models that could have been included in many more chapters than currently presented. We have done this on purpose – we have not written a book that is dedicated to any one behaviour or any one approach. We obviously cannot compete with more narrowly focused texts for specific behaviours or models. However, we present an overview with a thematic connection between the chapters which we hope readers will find interesting, thought provoking and, most importantly, of practical use.

We should also discuss why we have selected these topics for inclusion. On the one hand we could simply have discussed those mentioned by Tony Blair in his 2006 speech: 'obesity, smoking, alcohol abuse, . . . , sexually transmitted disease', but we recognised that this did not cover the complete range of behaviours we wanted to discuss. We initially included sleep as a lifestyle behaviour and thought that it was of key importance with the emergence (or, in reality, continued presence) of the 24-hour society and the increasing proportion of individuals involved in shift work. However, we came to realise that this did not fit with the other behaviours described in this text, so we abandoned this chapter. We then reviewed those behaviours which have the most significant impact on health and went for the chapters presented in this final volume.

Chapter 1: Introduction to healthy behaviour

In this opening chapter we set the context within which health practitioners are working and individuals are making choices about how they behave. We look historically at the socio-cultural climate in which we all operate, considering how and why lifestyle diseases and related behaviours have become so pertinent for us in the twenty-first century. We also consider the political imperative to encourage individual responsibility for long-term health and we reflect on the environmental influences over twenty-first century lifestyles.

Chapter 2: Psychology in practice

In this chapter we describe a number of key psychological concepts that are of relevance to the topic of lifestyle and lifestyle change. There are a great many theories of behavioural change, many of which include similar psychological concepts in different theoretical frameworks. The decision not to introduce specific theories but rather to introduce the key concepts that have consistently proved relevant for behavioural change is an attempt to bridge the gap between theory and practice. It is intended to make identifying the key aspects of research relevant to practice simpler. However, this is in no way intended to undermine the importance of theory, and the chapter highlights further reading that will enable interested readers to gain greater insight into the psychological theory that underpins these concepts. The existence of a large number of theories of behavioural change has been beneficial to our understanding of how and why people change their behaviour. It has enabled us to identify and understand those factors we might have expected to be important but are not, and those factors that are important in behavioural choices. However, it does make exploring the psychological research into behavioural change somewhat daunting for non-psychologists, so this chapter hopes to make the key psychological concepts to date easier to identify.

Chapter 3: Eating well

In this chapter we explore eating and diet. The problems in providing a clear message of a 'healthy diet' are stressed, as are the issues surrounding the social environment impact on diet. The governmental approaches to the 'obesity epidemic' are outlined and the role of psychological models in the development of appropriate interventions is stressed – ultimately, what the healthcare professional can do to promote healthy eating in those who are currently overweight, and how healthy eating can be promoted in the young.

Chapter 4: Being active

In this chapter we consider the predominance of sedentary lifestyles in the population. Physical activity is the output side of the input-output energy equation and so is a key factor in the rising levels of obesity. The role of the obesogenic environment and how psychological interventions can work in such adverse environmental conditions are explored.

Chapter 5: Sensible drinking

Drinking is a popular component of many aspects of leisure in Britain. Drinking has adverse consequences for social and physical well-being. The changing nature of drinking patterns in the UK and in particular in women is described and discussed. Government policies to establish healthy drinking patterns in the young and promote healthy drinking in adults are outlined and the role of psychological interventions to support healthy drinking and deter deleterious drinking is evaluated.

Chapter 6: Quitting smoking

The health consequences of smoking are well established and well known throughout the population - smoking can have a significant impact on morbidity and mortality. However, approximately a quarter of the population still smokes and this has a significant impact on both the individual and the country's health. Given the significant impact that smoking has on the health of the nation, there has been extensive research into smoking and much of this has a psychological nature. In this chapter, the psychological variables and models that have been applied to smoking and, more importantly, how they can be used to promote smoking cessation are discussed.

Chapter 7: Safer sex

The safe sex message is being promoted in order to reduce the spread of sexually transmitted diseases. Sexual behaviours are not simply a consequence of physiological drives, but there are social, emotional and cultural (to name but three) variables that influence such behaviour. Within these broader influences the psychological factors have to be appreciated and developed. These psychological models and how they can be applied to promote safer sex are discussed. Importantly, safer sex is discussed within a pleasure-promoting context rather than a fear-inducing one.

Chapter 8: Stopping illicit drug use

Illicit drug use is perhaps different from the other lifestyle behaviours explored in this text. It is a relatively rare behaviour but it has a clear impact on the community and the country at large. Furthermore, when exploring government material and recent academic texts, many include this as a lifestyle *choice* (although we acknowledge the debate around the use of the C-word). It is also important to recognise that illicit drug use can be categorised as a sub-category of smoking and alcohol abuse. The interventions designed to reduce illicit drug taking by employing psychological approaches which are relevant and essential to other lifestyle behaviours are discussed.

Chapter 9: Conclusion

This final chapter attempts to draw together the diverse behaviours discussed in the previous chapters and identify the key similarities and differences in the various behaviours we have considered. It is crucial for health practitioners to recognise which psychological techniques are effective across all behaviours in order to enable them to deal more effectively with the various prevention and promotion targets they are required to meet. This final chapter also tries to look ahead and identify what else we need to know to make our interventions more effective.

For each of these chapters we have included a selection of the following features:

- *Learning objectives:* What you will find in this book, so that you can navigate your way through the text and know what to expect and what you can achieve.
- *Case study:* We provide a brief case study that highlights some key principles to be discussed later in the chapter. In some of these you are asked to take the role of the individual practitioner dealing with the client and we hope that this will highlight issues that you may face in practice (or have faced), whether this be as a qualified or student healthcare professional. We hope that the case study will raise questions and issues that we address later in the chapter.
- *Introduction:* The introduction follows the case study – we hope that the case study has whetted your appetite and you will begin to appreciate during the chapter the importance of the case study and how it relates to the chapter content.
- *Key messages:* These key points are littered throughout the chapter, highlighting the key messages that are in the text.
- *Applying this to. . . :* At stages throughout the chapter a box highlights how the principles discussed in the text can be applied to the case study.
- *Discussion points:* These act as points for discussion – they relate either to all of the chapter content or to the case study highlighted at the outset.
- *Applying research in practice:* In the chapter, empirical research studies are presented throughout to demonstrate the evidence base of the suggested techniques. More detail on a couple of these is provided in these boxes.
- *Putting this into action:* A final box at the end of the chapter contains all of the principles and skills discussed during the chapter and finally applies it to the case study.

We hope you are interested and engaged in this book and that it leads to an enhancement of your personal and professional skills. Overall, we hope that it leads to an improvement in healthy behaviours in your client group and goes some way to reducing the immense health problems associated with a poor lifestyle currently evident in the UK today.

References

Blair, T. (2006). Speech on healthy living. *The Guardian*, 26 July. Available at: http://www.guardian.co.uk/society/2006/jul/26/health.politics (accessed 30 November 2009).

Jones, A., Bentham, G., Foster, C., Hillsdon, M. and Panter, J. (2007). *Tackling Obesities: Future Choices - Obesogenic Environments - Evidence Review*. London: United Kingdom Government Foresight Programme, Office of Science and Innovation.

Liddle, R. (2008). Laugh at the lard butts - but just remember Fatty Fritz lives longer. *Sunday Times*, 27 January.

Thirlaway, K. and Upton, D. (2009). *The Psychology of Lifestyle:* Promoting Healthy Behaviour. London: Routledge.

Acknowledgements

Author acknowledgements

Both of us have spent considerable time on this project, collating, reading and reviewing research articles and textbooks before trying to develop the material into a series of practical chapters that could assist and develop an individual professional's practice. The material we have read has not only been presented by psychologists but also by those from the wider academic community, including those from healthcare, medicine, sociology, philosophy and policy developments. We have tried to encompass the literature from both an academic and a practitioner basis. We thank the researchers, clinicians and policy makers for all this work and the contributions they have made to the current knowledge base.

On a more personal level, several key colleagues have acted as researchers and reviewers for us and have contributed their time, effort and opinions with vigour and a frankness that was as refreshing as it was useful. Particular mention should go to Erica Thomas and Julia Mathias (for DU) and Jemma Hawkins and Kath John (for KT).

Many thanks also to the team at Pearson's Higher Education Division for helping us through this project. Finally, we also thank those involved in the production of this text – the designers and production editors – for enhancing the text with some excellent features, which we hope will provide guidance, direction and added value to all readers.

We must also offer thanks and acknowledgements to those who have provided support for us both at work and at home. We also thank our colleagues (for DU) at the University of Worcester and (for KT) at the University of Wales Institute, Cardiff (UWIC) for their help, advice, friendship and practical guidance.

Finally, we would like to thank our family and friends for bringing us sustenance and calming us down during our manic periods. In particular, our children: Dominic's children – Francesca, Rosie and Gabriel (my favourite) and Katie's children – Anna, Hetty and Keir. As always, Katie would not have been able to complete the book without the support of Megan and Sue.

Publisher acknowledgements

We are grateful to the following for permission to reproduce copyright material:

Figures

Figure 3.3 adapted from 'In search of how people change: applications to addictive behaviors', American Psychologist, 47(9), pp. 1102–1114 (Prochaska, J.O., DiClemente, C.C. and Norcross, J.C. 1992), *American Psychiatric Association*, adapted with permission; Figure 4.1

from *The psychology of lifestyle: promoting healthy behaviour*, Routledge (Thirlaway, K.J. and Upton, D. 2009), with permission from Taylor & Francis Books (UK); Figure 4.2 adapted from *Tackling obesities: future choices – obsofenic environments – evidence review*, Government Office for Science (Jones, A., Bentham., G. Foster, C., Hillsdon, M. and Panter, J. 2007), © Crown copyright 2007. Reproduced under the terms of the Click-Use Licence; Figure 6.2 adapted from National Institute for Clinical Health and Clinical Excellence (2006), *PH1 Brief interventions and referral for smoking cessation in primary and other settings*. London: NICE (2006). Available from www.nice.org.uk/PH1. Reproduced with permission; Figure 6.3 adapted from © Silverman, Jonathan and Draper, Juliet, *Skills for Communicating with Patients* 2nd edn. Oxford: Radcliffe Publishing, 2005. Adapted from the original work by Prochaska and DiClemente (1986). Reproduced with the permission of the copyright holder; Figure 7.2 from *Sexual behaviour in Britain: the national survey of sexual attitudes and lifestyles* (© J. Fields, J. Wadsworth, A. Johnson, K. Wellings, 1994). Reproduced by permission of PFD (www.pfd.co.uk); Figure 7.3 adapted with kind permission from Springer Science and Business Media, 'Promoting condom use with main partners: a behavioural intervention trail for women', *AIDS and Behaviour*, 5, 193–204 (Gielen, A.C., Fogarty, L.A., Armstrong, K., Green, B.M., Cabral, R., Milstein, B., Galavotti, C., and Heilig, C.M. 2001); Figure 8.1 from *International Classification of Diseases*, available at http://www.who.int/classifications/ apps/icd/icd20online/, 10 rev., World Health Organization (WHO 2007a) WHO. Reproduced with permission.

Tables

Table 2.3 and 6.10 adapted from *Motivational interviewing: Preparing people for change*, 2nd edn., Guilford Press (Miller, W.R. and Rollnick, S. 2002). Reproduced with permission; Table 3.1 from *Annex 7 – Impact Assessment Consultation on Television Advertising of Food and Drink to Children*. Joint FSA/DoH Analysis, 2 (2006) © Ofcom copyright 2006; Table 4.2 adapted from *At least 5 a day a week*, Department of Health (Department of Health 2004) © Crown copyright 2004. Crown copyright material is reproduced with permission under the terms of the Click-Use Licence; Table 5.5 from *Safe. Sensible. Social. The Next Steps in the National Alchohol Strategy*, Department of Health and The Home Office (2007), © Crown copyright 2007. Reproduced under the terms of the Click-Use Licence; Tables 5.7, 9.1 adapted from *Public Health Ethical Issues*, Nuffield Council on Bioethics, Available at: www.nuffield bioethics.org (Nuffield Council on Bioethics 2007), adapted with permission; Table 6.4 adapted from *British Medical Journal*, 328, pp. 338–39 (West, R. 2004) with permission from BMJ Publishing Group Ltd.; Table 6.6 adapted from 'Interventions to facilitate smoking cessation', *American Family Physician*, 74, 262–71 (Okuyemi, K.S., Nollen, N.L. and Ahluwalia, J.S. 2006), adapted with permission; Table 6.8 adapted from 'Relapse to smoking', *Clinical Psychology Review*, 26(2), pp. 196–215, (Piasecki, T.) Copyright 2006, with permission from Elsevier; Table 6.12 reproduced from *British Medical Journal*, 328, pp. 277–79 (Jarvis, Martin J. 2004), with permission from BMJ Publishing Group Ltd.; Table 7.3 from *All new episodes seen at GUM clinics: 1998–2007. United Kingdom and country specific tables* (Health Protection Agency 2008), Copyright Health Protection Agency, reproduced with permission; Table 7.4 *Reprinted from Journal of Adolescent Health, 40 (1), Eric R. Buhi and Patricia Goodson*, Predictors of adolescent and sexual behaviour and intention: A theory-guided systematic review, *4–21, Copyright 2007, with permission from Elsevier*; Tables 8.3, 8.4 from *Crime in England and Wales 2006/7*, 4th edn., Home Office (Nicholas, S., Kershaw, C. and Walker, K. (eds) 2008), © Crown copyright 2008. Reproduced under the terms of the Click-Use Licence;

Table 8.5 from 'Drug-related poisoning deaths: by selected type of drug, 1993 to 2000', *Social Trends*, 33 ed. (ONS 2005), © Crown Copyright 2005. Reproduced under the terms of the Click-Use Licence; Table 8.9 adapted from *Estimating the prevalence of problematic and injecting drug use for Drug Action Team areas in England: a feasibility study using the Multiple Indicator Method*. Home Office online report 34/04, available at http://www.homeoffice.gov.uk/rds/pdfs04/rdsolr2404.pdf, Home Office (Frischer, M., Heatlie, H. and Hickman, M. 2004), © Crown copyright 2009. Reproduced under the terms of the Click-Use Licence; Table 8.11 from *Risk, protective factors and resilience to drug use: identifying resilient young people and learning from their experience*, Home Office (Dillon, L., Chivite-Matthews, N., Grewal, I., Brown, R., Webster, S., Weddell, E., Brown, G. and Smith, N. (2007)) Home Office, © Crown copyright 2007. Reproduced under the terms of the Click-Use Licence.

Photographs

The publisher would like to thank the following for their kind permission to reproduce their photographs:

Photographs 2.1 and 2.2 from The Advertising Archives; Photograph 2.3 © DOHMH; Photograph 2.4 © European Union, 2010; Photograph 3.1 from Food Standards Agency, http://www.eatwell.gov.uk/healthydiet/eatwellplate/?lang=en, © Crown copyright 2007. Reproduced under the terms of the Click-Use Licence.

In some instances we have been unable to trace the owners of copyright material, and we would appreciate any information that would enable us to do so.

Chapter 1
Introduction to healthy behaviour

LEARNING OBJECTIVES

At the end of this chapter you will:

- Recognise how the concepts of lifestyle diseases and lifestyle behaviours have arisen
- Understand the health behaviours central to the development and progression of chronic diseases
- Recognise why lifestyle change is so complex and difficult
- Recognise the multiple influences on lifestyle choice
- Understand the challenges for health professionals involved in health promotion

Health professionals and particularly primary care practitioners have health promotion and disease prevention as a central aspect of their role. This book is about this central element of a healthcare professional's role. Although lifestyle change should be a key part of *all* health professionals' role, and this has been recognised for many decades, in recent years its importance has moved higher up the policy hierarchy. For example, the then prime minister of the UK, Tony Blair, in 2006 called for 'lifestyle change' to relieve the pressure on the National Health Service (BBC News, 2006): the prime minister suggested that 'failure to address bad lifestyles was putting an "increasing strain" on the health service'. The impact of this key message, the role of lifestyle in health, has been significant. Many health professionals now provide the patients and clients who come into their clinics with expert advice about lifestyle behaviours and health. The frustration and disillusionment that are felt when advice is ignored and patients go on to develop chronic diseases that could probably have been avoided are among the motivating factors for this book. This frustration is frequently articulated by health professionals involved in treating the major lifestyle diseases of the twentieth century. In 2009, Professor Wiseman, medical and scientific adviser for the World Cancer Research Fund, said:

> *This means that we are now more sure than ever before that by limiting the amount of alcohol they drink, maintaining a healthy weight and being physically active women can*

make a significant difference to their risk. We estimate over 40% of breast cancer cases in the UK could be prevented just by making these relatively straightforward changes.

Wiseman (2009)

Lifestyle change is a tantalising solution to the chronic ill-health that is the scourge of modern societies. It is such a cheap, effective, non-toxic, low-risk solution to the rising incidence of heart disease, diabetes, chronic back pain, cancers and many other conditions that it can seem incredible that we have not been able to deliver widespread population change. This book does not present a method to effect instant population-wide uptake of health advice but it does explain why changing lifestyle behaviours is so difficult for so many people and not quite as straightforward as Professor Wiseman suggests. Furthermore this book points the reader in the direction of techniques and interventions proven to have at least some success in increasing the likelihood of successful behavioural change.

So what are the key health behaviours that the government would like us to change? The word lifestyle is used confidently by health professionals, the media and individuals but what does it mean and which health behaviours are included under its umbrella? Initially, the medical profession started to refer to 'lifestyle diseases' to reflect the role that lifestyle choices play in certain diseases. Doyle (2001) suggested that the six major lifestyle diseases are coronary heart disease, stroke, lung cancer, colon cancer, diabetes and chronic obstructive pulmonary disease. The rationale for their inclusion is that they 'trace mainly to imprudent living' (Doyle, 2001).

Interestingly, few authors would call sexually transmitted diseases 'lifestyle diseases', although they are clearly entirely a result of behavioural choices with none of the genetic component that plays a part in the six major lifestyle diseases identified by Doyle (2001). Sexually transmitted diseases are more usually defined as infectious diseases (ONS, 2007), an important distinction for clinicians but perhaps less so for primary care and community-based practitioners interested in public health.

In between an 'imprudent lifestyle' (Doyle, 2001) and the development of lifestyle diseases are a number of 'precursor' conditions. High cholesterol, high blood pressure and obesity are risk factors for the development of a number of the aforementioned lifestyle diseases. The distinction between these precursors, the diseases they predict and the behaviours that are associated with them is often blurred. They are often presented as diseases *per se* and interventions are prescribed by the medical profession. The Department of Health (1999) categorises high blood pressure as a cardiovascular disease. Obesity is frequently referred to using disease parameters. For instance, the phrase 'obesity epidemic' (Gard and Wright, 2005) is common and suggests that obesity is a disease and furthermore that it is somehow catching! Consequently, obesity is considered a lifestyle disease by some authors whereas others categorise it as lifestyle behaviour (Doyle, 2001).

The behaviours that are usually cited as being involved in the aetiology of lifestyle diseases are poor diet, lack of physical activity, cigarette smoking (Doyle, 2001; Blaxter, 1990) and, increasingly, excess drinking (Burke *et al.*, 1997; Blaxter, 1990). The taking of illegal drugs is also a lifestyle behaviour with health consequences. However, drug takers, whilst often high profile, currently constitute a minority of the population and so reducing illegal drug taking seldom appears in general government health targets. Drug taking may be an issue only for a minority but nevertheless it is essentially the same behaviour as smoking and drinking, with the added social consequences and implications of being illegal. The taking of certain illegal drugs remains a serious problem in the UK and Europe (European

Monitoring Centre for Drugs and Drug Addiction, accessed 2009) and consequently illegal drug taking is included in this text.

Sexual practices are also often described by public health professionals as health and/or lifestyle behaviours (Wardle and Steptoe, 2005). Despite not being directly linked to what clinicians refer to as lifestyle diseases, sexual practices nevertheless are still considered by most public health practitioners to be an aspect of lifestyle worthy of both concern and intervention (Wardle and Steptoe, 2005). Furthermore, sexual practices are a clear cause of preventable and treatable diseases. Consequently, the promotion of safer sex is also included in this book.

Over the past couple of decades the unhealthy lifestyles that predominate in Western societies have been presented by the media as a new and modern crisis. Stories about drunken young women, rising levels of obesity and type 2 diabetes are no longer restricted to the health pages but frequently take the front pages of national papers and make the lead story of television news bulletins. However, it is important to recognise that people have been drinking too much and eating the wrong things for many centuries. In Victorian times there were many gin addicts and in Elizabethan times diets were poor and dangerous levels of drinking were widespread (Plant and Plant, 2006). Perhaps the main difference between then and now is the level of understanding we have. We have a better understanding of the relationship between our lifestyle and our health than previous generations. However, as long ago as Roman times, the importance of a moderate lifestyle was recognised. For example, Pythagoras suggests that 'No man, who values his health, ought to trespass on the bounds of moderation, either in labour, diet or concubinage' and Hippocrates that 'Persons of a gross relaxed habit of body, the flabby, and red-haired, ought to use a drying diet . . . Such as are fat, and desire to be lean, should use exercise fasting; should drink small liquors a little warm, should eat only once a day, and no more than will just satisfy their hunger' (cited in Haslam, 2007, p. 32). The connection between obesity and angina was emphasised in 1811 by Robert Thomas who wrote: 'It is found to attack men much more frequently than women, particularly those who have short necks, who are inclinable to corpulency, and who at the same time lead an inactive or sedentary life . . . he should endeavor to counteract disposition to obesity, which has been considered a predisposing cause' (Thomas, 1811).

It was towards the end of the eighteenth and during the nineteenth century that lifestyle approaches to health in Western societies were subsumed in the battle to control infectious diseases. Developing industrial societies and their new, crowded, urban ways of living promoted the spread of infectious diseases such as smallpox, scarlet fever etc. (Scambler, 2003). In reality, better sanitation, nutrition and living conditions led to the decline of infectious diseases, but at the same time as these public health measures were being instigated, doctors were simultaneously starting to understand that diseases such as smallpox and measles were caused by single infectious agents. Vaccines were developed against these and people were protected from the associated diseases. Antibiotics to treat bacterial infections were discovered and on the back of these major discoveries the biomedical principle that all disease can be traced to specific causal mechanisms emerged and dominated the practice and development of medicine over the next century (Scambler, 2003). Many would argue that the biomedical model of disease still remains the underlying principle behind the majority of medical practice in Western societies. However, in actuality, a number of models of disease and health (such as genetic, environmental and lifestyle models) influence medical practice and public health initiatives; it is just that the biomedical model usually takes prominence.

Infectious diseases have declined throughout the twentieth and twenty-first centuries and in some cases have been completely eradicated. The major health problems for modern developed societies are the chronic or so-called 'lifestyle diseases' identified by Doyle (2001). These chronic conditions are complex and cannot easily be traced to specific causal mechanisms. They are influenced at a number of levels – biologically, psychologically and sociologically. That is to say, the genes we inherit and the environment we inhabit are central to whether we go on to develop a chronic disease. Pivotal to the genetic and environmental circumstances of an individual is the way they respond to their environment and to their biological make-up. One individual may recognise that diabetes 'runs' in their family and make active choices to try to prevent it. Another with the same understanding of their family history may decide that it is inevitable that they will develop the disease and continue with damaging health choices. Similarly, one person may use smoking as a coping strategy to deal with the adverse environmental circumstances they find themselves in whereas the next may use exercise as a coping strategy. In this text we recognise that the socio-cultural circumstances in which an individual finds themselves can severely limit their lifestyle choices but we argue that usually some level of choice remains. This text explores how to encourage positive lifestyle change whilst recognising that the biological and environmental circumstances of each individual will vary enormously and have a large role to play in the degree of volitional choice each person has.

The biomedical model of disease is often characterised as curative but also has a preventative remit, albeit one that is frequently focused on vaccination or the avoidance of a specific causal organism. Chronic diseases are not generally something that you catch; rather they are a long-term response to stressors such as poor diet, lack of exercise, excess alcohol, high blood pressure, poverty or environmental hazards. Consequently, the lifestyle model of disease, first promoted by the Greeks/Romans, is once again taking precedence and influencing health policy.

A lifestyle model of disease is very focused on prevention. Lifestyle changes are clearly still pertinent once a disease is diagnosed and can slow the progress of the disease and reduce complications, but fundamentally the principle of lifestyle change is to prevent disease. This can be viewed as a threat to the medical profession and to commercial companies that make a profit from curing disease. However, lifestyle approaches have their own commercial spin-offs and the proliferation of private gyms and diet products is a visible sign of the commercial potential of a lifestyle approach to health and disease prevention.

Lifestyle approaches to health, whilst having the potential to generate profit for commercial operators, are attractive to governments because of the potential to shift the responsibility for health from the government to the individual. In this way, whilst some can see a way to profit from lifestyle approaches to health, the government can see a potential low-cost solution to healthcare. Many policy documents emphasise the role of individual choice in health-related behaviour and stress personal responsibility. There is a danger that this approach can be seen as a 'way out' for governments who can fairly cheaply provide individuals with the information they need to make informed choices about their lifestyle and leave them to get on with it. However, this is a short-sighted approach because when such tactics don't work the NHS is still 'burdened' with the job of treating people who have developed chronic diseases. Indeed, many commentators remain concerned about the lifestyle approach to disease, arguing that by emphasising individual choice the huge social factors involved in inequities in health can be ignored.

It is certainly true that early responses to the evidence that chronic diseases are influenced by behaviour did focus on knowledge-based health promotion campaigns that left the individual to resolve any behavioural flaws. However, the evidence from decades of educational health promotion is that it doesn't produce lifestyle change. Recently, public health policy makers at all levels have made position statements about expanding the medical definition of 'lifestyle' to take into account the social nature of lifestyle behaviour (Ashton and Seymour, 1988; Bruce, 1991; Armstong, 1993, cited in Hansen and Easthope, 2007). 'New public health', as it has been described, aims to discard health education initiatives in favour of enhancing people's life skills and creating supportive environments (McPearson, 1992; Ashton and Seymour, 1988). 'New public health' operates with a biopsychosocial understanding of health which requires education and lifestyle modification to be part of general public policy, the workplace and education, not restricted to health promotional campaigns (O'Conner and Parker, 1995, cited in Hansen and Easthope, 2007). The lifestyle model of disease, rather than being individualistic, can at its best enable individuals to take control of their health and influence policy to enable them to do so. The importance of supportive environments in promoting behavioural change has been emphasised recently by the impressive impact of the public smoking ban on rates of heart attacks, reduced by 10% in England and 14% in Scotland (Nursing Times, accessed 2009).

If we are to move away from a health promotion approach to lifestyle behaviour towards developing people's 'life skills' then a sound basis in the psychology of behavioural change will be necessary. To move from providing knowledge to improving the ability to change requires a psychological approach. We need to work with people within their current socio-economic resources whilst pressurising governments to provide the resources to enable change.

As recognised by the World Health Organisation (1986), lifestyle is more than simply an individual choice. The way we live is dictated by our economic and cultural circumstances (Blaxter, 1990). Indeed, the use of the term 'lifestyle change' reflects the importance of socio-demographic factors in health behaviour change rather better than the term 'health promotion'. Ethnicity, sex, age, socio-economic circumstances and cultural groups all interplay to influence the way we choose to behave (Blaxter, 1990). The evidence for socio-demographic influences on lifestyle choices is irrefutable (Craig and Mindell, 2008).

The UK government and more recently the devolved institutions of Wales, Scotland and Northern Ireland have been collecting demographic mortality and morbidity data for some time, enabling comparisons between the health of different demographic and socio-economic groups. More recently, data on physical activity, eating habits, drinking and smoking have also been included. Each of these UK institutions has commissioned surveys on a continuing basis to enable comparisons between behaviours over time and to monitor health targets. The demographic data collected in each survey includes sex, age and socio-economic class. Each of these will be explored in the coming section to detail how these demographic factors can influence health and well-being so that the healthcare professional is able to recognise and understand the influence that some of these variables exert.

Both biological sex and gender are related to health and health outcomes, but it is generally accepted that it is gender rather than biological sex that influences lifestyle choices. Indeed, the gender influence on health is primarily mediated through lifestyle choices. Many studies confuse the terms sex and gender. Sex is the biological underpinning – our genetic make-up. Gender, on the other hand, is socially constructed; it is more concerned with how we think and behave (Annandale and Hunt, 2000).

A woman born in 2007 has a life expectancy of 84 years, a man only 77 years (ONS, 2007). Men and women also have different morbidity rates. For example, women are less likely to suffer from cardiovascular disease and more likely to suffer from breast cancer than men (ONS, 2007). Prostate cancer is a solely male disease as women do not have a prostate gland. Male and female differences in morbidity and mortality are influenced by biological sex (physiological and hormonal differences) but also by gender and gender role casting (Annandale and Hunt, 2000). The difference in male and female mortality rates is diminishing and this is generally held to be due to changing gender roles in Western societies rather than to biological factors, although early menarche may play a part in the rising prevalence of some female hormonally-linked cancers. Unfortunately, not all gender role adaptations are positive and some of these changes in gender expectations have resulted in women adopting unhealthy, traditionally male lifestyle behaviours (Emslie *et al.*, 2002). The influence of gender over health is mediated through the lifestyle choices that men and women make. The implications of gender roles for the various lifestyle behaviours will be developed and discussed in the relevant chapters.

Age is different from every other demographic variable in that the majority of us will experience old age. There are clear differences in health and health outcomes between different age categories and, unlike sex/gender differences, a large factor will be physiological changes over the lifespan rather than cultural expectations about age-related behaviour. Nevertheless, cultural expectations of how people of different ages should behave do play a role in the way that, for example, teenage mothers approach their pregnancies and older people participate in exercise and sport. Furthermore, despite the fact that presumably we must all hope to become older, older people experience considerable discrimination, which has implications for their health and well-being and for their lifestyle choices (Scambler, 2003). Hence, it is important to explore the impact of the cultural influences of age on lifestyle and health and this will be addressed in each of the lifestyle behaviour chapters.

Socio-economic is a broad term encompassing many variables and is assessed using a range of different factors. Social class, income, work, housing, physical and social environments have all been found to influence our health directly and also indirectly through their influence on lifestyle choices (Doyle, 2001). The definition of social class adopted by this text has been provided by the seminal Black Report (Townsend and Davidson, 1989) which first clearly stated the link between health and social class in modern society:

> *Segments of the population sharing broadly similar types and levels of resources, with broadly similar styles of living and (for some sociologists), some shared perception of their collective condition.*

In essence, different classes have differential power to access material resources: homes, cars, white and electronic goods etc.

Explanations for behavioural choices are both contentious and politically sensitive. In 1989 Townsend and Davidson recognised that there were a number of explanations for differing levels of health in different sections of society. The key most plausible explanations are a materialist explanation and a behavioural explanation. Simply, a materialist explanation suggests that most of the class differences in health can be explained by the environmental circumstances in which individuals find themselves. A behavioural explanation suggests that most of the class differences in health can be explained by the choices that individuals make. At first sight, these explanations would seem to argue for different causes of disease but actually the distinction is more subtle. To use late-onset diabetes as an example, a behaviourist explanation would argue that a proportion of the class difference in diabetes morbidity can be explained by what individuals choose to eat. A materialist explanation does not refute the claim that diet is a major cause of late-onset diabetes but questions the degree of choice that individuals actually have about the food that they eat. Another way of framing the dichotomy is in terms of individual or collective responsibility. In the first case, the right of individuals to do as they wish with their own lives is emphasised; in the second, the inability of individuals to exert control over their environment is considered key (Blaxter, 1990). At first sight, a lifestyle model of health would appear to operate within behaviourist or individualistic explanations for lifestyle choices. However, for these authors the use of the term lifestyle behaviours rather than health behaviours is a deliberate attempt to recognise the role of socio-environmental factors in decisions individuals make about behaviours that impinge on their health. The challenge for health practitioners is to identify how to enable individuals to make positive changes to their lifestyle within the socio-economic circumstances in which they live in. In other words, it is hoped that recognising that social and environmental circumstances are an integral aspect of lifestyle choice does not rule out the possibility of effective behavioural change within those parameters. Clearly, a blanket-style approach to lifestyle change is unlikely to be successful and lifestyle interventions must be tailored to the circumstances in which individuals find themselves.

One popular way of describing the role of the environment in behavioural choice is to refer to obesogenic environments. The common use of the term obesogenic environment reflects the widening acceptance of the role of factors external to the individual in the development of obesity. The complexities of what contributes to an obesogenic environment are not well understood. We know that roads and cars promote sedentary modes of travel through their ease and convenience and discourage active transport by being a danger to pedestrians and cyclists, but cars also enable people to travel to leisure activities that support health and well-being. We understand that the easy availability of high-calorie food and the increasing portion size in restaurants promote over-eating of the 'wrong' types of food but there is far greater availability of healthy food choices as well. Other factors such as shift working, alcohol and drug consumption, media output etc. all contribute to an obesogenic environment. The key to what makes an environment obesogenic would seem to be understanding and influencing the cultural responses we make to that environment (Jones *et al.*, 2007).

Lifestyle behaviours have multiple functions; they are not simply or even primarily health focused. Lifestyle behaviours play a key role in developing and maintaining social relationships. They can be mood enhancing or a way of coping with stressful circumstances. Lifestyle behaviours are often pleasurable. Furthermore, the roles they play in our lives change during the lifespan. Lifestyle behaviours are all under some degree of volitional control, although the amount of control individuals have over their lifestyle choices is debatable and likely to vary a lot between people. The term lifestyle reflects that these are behaviours we do regularly and probably habitually. Lifestyle behaviours have the majority of their positive consequences in the present and the majority of their negative outcomes in the future. Any lifestyle behavioural change intervention consequently requires individuals to be future orientated. When you start to consider the complexity of lifestyle behaviours it becomes apparent why change is not as straightforward as it first appears.

It is true that, to some extent, the rise in chronic diseases is actually a reflection of the success of modern healthcare and social reform in that more people live long enough to experience the chronic conditions associated with old age. However, there is considerable evidence that, in addition, people take less exercise (Department of Health, 2004), drink more alcohol (HM Government, 2007), are less safe in their sexual practices (Center for Disease Control, 2007), are more likely to take illegal drugs (ONS, 2007) and eat poorer diets (Fox and Hillsdon, 2007) than they did in previous recent generations. Smoking is the only lifestyle behaviour where incidence is declining, although a considerable minority of the population continue to smoke (ONS, 2007). It is important to try to understand why unhealthy lifestyles have become so widespread, particularly since Western societies seem to be exporting these deleterious practices to developing nations (WHO, 1986).

The lifestyles of societies are constantly evolving and will change in response to modernisation and social reform. We can see this in the different patterns of lifestyle choices in countries at different stages of modernisation and with different cultural norms (WHO, 1986). Life in modernised societies is easier and requires less physical effort than it did in previous generations (Department of Health, 2004; Fox and Hillsdon, 2007). Employment is more likely to be sedentary, housework is less demanding and far fewer people are physically active in the process of travelling. There is no evidence that people are less active in their leisure time than they were in previous generations but because the majority of physical activity is now leisure, people's total physical activity has declined (Department of Health, 2004). The increase in cheap fast-food outlets, high-calorie snacks and ready-prepared meals all contribute to the poorer diets we eat today (Myslobodsky, 2003). Alcohol has become considerably cheaper than it was in previous generations and is more readily available (Plant and Plant, 2006; Babor et al., 2003). Cultural acceptance of heavy drinking remains a stable facet of British life but a key change here is that it used to be unacceptable for young women to drink heavily; however, changing gender expectations are making it more acceptable for young women to match young men in their excessive drinking (Plant and Plant, 2006). It is probably in terms of sexual behaviour that cultural expectations have altered most dramatically, with sex outside marriage and children out of wedlock virtually normalised in secular society (Schubotz et al., 2003). There are many positives from a more liberal attitude towards sex. It has enabled better education and communication about safe sex, empowering some women to control their sexual destinies and consequently protect themselves from sexual infection and unwanted pregnancy.

Beck (1990) coined the phrase 'risk society' to acknowledge that we live in a world where perceptions of risk are heightened, and the identification and management of risk are a major concern at all levels of society. Risk assessment in the workplace is now a legal requirement. Similarly, in schools and colleges all activities must be risk assessed, which may result in a reduction of school trips if procedures to mitigate the risk cannot be simply and cheaply instigated. Alongside risk assessment has emerged the concept of informed consent. Many professionals, health practitioners included, must ensure that they have the informed consent of an individual before embarking on a treatment programme or other intervention. All these procedures combine to create the impression that we live in a high-risk environment, when in reality we are probably safer from environmental hazards and disease than at any previous point in history. The perception of a high-risk environment is further perpetuated by the media who bombard us with 'risk' stories. Stories about crime, environmental and health risks dominate the media because they meet key news agendas in that they are negative and often sensational: 'Drinking a glass of wine a day increases your risk of breast cancer by 6%'. Lifestyle risks such as the risk of breast cancer from alcohol consumption are just some of a range of risks that we need to manage daily. For many people the best way to deal with the plethora of risk messages that they receive on a daily basis is to ignore them (Thirlaway and Heggs, 2005).

Lifestyle behaviours are embedded in daily life. There are four aspects to most people's lives: sleeping, travelling, occupation and leisure (Buckworth and Dishman, 2002). However, it is impossible to describe a typical 24 hours for someone working in the UK. The complexities of modern life in terms of work patterns and outside responsibilities mean that fewer and fewer people work a nine to five day. However, if you consider an average night's sleep to be about eight hours, the average working day to be eight hours and an average journey to and from work to be an hour then there are about seven hours left a day for leisure and/or caring and household responsibilities. Obviously, many people will take longer to travel to work, sleep for longer or less, have greater or fewer responsibilities outside of work, but most people will have some time each day that is not taken up with travelling, work, caring or sleeping. Many people do not work for longer than eight hours at a time. People in the UK work some of the longest hours in Europe and also many people work fewer but longer days each week, e.g. those in the police force and nursing. Shift work is common and it is associated with unhealthy lifestyle choices (Folkhard et al., 2005). Probably one of the major changes in daily living in the UK has been the huge increase in parents with young children who work (ONS, 2007). This means that people are busy with household responsibilities outside of work that may previously have been completed during the day. In summary, given that the physically active nature of housework and shopping has reduced (Department of Health, 2004) and that there has been a reduction in time available for physically active pursuits, it is not surprising that changes in the pattern of a 'normal' day have had consequences for both lifestyle and health.

While we are travelling we could be physically active, we could eat or smoke. However, smoking has recently been banned in all public places, including public transport vehicles, in the UK. This is the first major piece of legislation for many years that pertains to volitional lifestyle behaviour and evidence is emerging that the public ban has had a significant positive effect on heart attack rates in the UK (Nursing Times, accessed 2009). Private cars are not subject to the legislation so it is possible that the ban may encourage people to use their cars if they wish to smoke on a journey, but there is no evidence yet of this.

For the majority of people the trip to work, school or college is the most frequent journey. A minority of people take the opportunity to walk or cycle to their place of work or study but the majority will drive or use public transport. Regular travel by foot or by bicycle has declined by 26% (Department of Health, 2004) over the past 20 to 30 years. Factors believed to contribute to the decline of regular travel by foot or bicycle include: perceived and actual safety; the provision of facilities to segregate conflicting road users; and the proximity of local shops/workplace (Jones et al., 2007).

Work and caring for relatives are the primary occupations for most people and the majority of jobs these days are predominantly sedentary (Department of Health, 2004). Similarly, most caring roles do not involve physical activity, although they can require heavy lifting. At work, most people will eat at least one meal and the quality of available food will influence the food choices. Jeffery et al. (2006) found no relationship between the proximity of fast-food outlets to the workplace and what people ate. There is little evidence about the influence of on-site food provision in the workplace on food choice, although the healthy workplace initiatives in Scotland (Scotland Health Improvement Agency, accessed 2009) and Wales (Welsh Assembly Government, accessed 2009) were designed to improve on-site food choice. The majority of work on on-site provision of food has been carried out with children. Previously, unhealthy food choices have dominated school food sales but the impact of new nutritional standards in schools in September 2006 is yet to be evaluated (Jones et al., 2007; see Chapters 3 on eating well).

Whilst drinking alcohol at work is extremely rare, the workplace culture of drinking outside of working hours has been found to be significantly related to both drinking with work colleagues and non-work-related drinking (Delaney and Ames, 1995; Barrientos-Gutierrez et al., 2007). The establishment of healthy drinking norms in the workplace could have beneficial effects for drinking both with work colleagues and more widely.

Patterns of leisure activity have changed dramatically with the development of sedentary activities such as watching television, using computers and the myriad of electronic games consoles available. The relationship between time spent in such sedentary leisure activities and reductions in time spent in physically active leisure pursuits has been, and still is, the subject of much concern, particularly in children (Department of Health, 2004). At the same time the number of health clubs and gyms has proliferated and a small increase in the proportion of people taking leisure-time physical activity has been reported (Department of Health, 2004). Television cookery programmes are popular but it would seem that watching cookery programmes rather than actually cooking is the popular leisure pursuit! Other popular leisure activities such as going to the cinema are associated with unhealthy food availability and large portion sizes. Similarly, recent studies have highlighted the increase in portion sizes of meals served in restaurants (Nielsen and Popkin, 2003). Hence, leisure activities themselves can lead to an increase in unhealthy lifestyles.

Conclusion

The world we live in is both the safest yet and a highly risky place, and probably the biggest risk to health, for most people, is the lifestyle choices that they make. However, most of us continue to be concerned about dramatic risks such as aeroplane crashes, but continue to ignore the far more likely risks associated with a lifetime of smoking, eating and drinking too much and remaining sedentary. Education has little impact on people's failure to respond to risk. Choices about eating, drinking, smoking or physical activity are possible, although not for everyone in every context. Enabling choice, supporting choice, empowering choice is what all health practitioners want to achieve, and understanding how best to do this is what this book is about.

Summary points

- The major lifestyle diseases are coronary heart disease, stroke, lung cancer, colon cancer, diabetes and chronic obstructive pulmonary disease.
- Unhealthy lifestyles have arisen as a response to modern society.
- We understand the risks associated with unhealthy lifestyle behaviours probably better than at any other time in history but still fail to make appropriate changes to our behaviour.
- Lifestyle change is more difficult for some people than others, depending on their socio-demographic and environmental circumstances.
- Lifestyle behaviours are complex, which makes instigating change similarly complex and difficult.

References

Annandale, E. and Hunt, K. (2000). *Gender Inequalities in Health*. Buckingham: Open University Press.

Ashton, J. and Seymour, H. (1988) *The New Public Health: The Liverpool Experience*. Milton Keynes: Open University Press.

Babor, T., Caetano, R., Casswell, S., Edwards, G., Giesbrecht, N., Graham, K., Grube, J., Gruenewald, P., Hill, L., Holder, H., Homel, R., Osterberg, E., Rehm, J., Room, R. and Rossow, I. (2003). *Alcohol: No Ordinary Commodity*. Oxford: Oxford University Press.

Barrientos-Gutierrez, T., Gimeno, D., Mangiane, T.W., Harrist, R.B. and Amick, B.C. (2007). Drinking social norms and drinking behaviours. *Occupational and Environmental Medicine*, 64, 602-608.

BBC. (2006). http://www.worcestershirehealth.nhs.uk/whs_recruitment/recruitment_waht/medical_dental/WD06_07.asp

Beck, U. (1990). *Risk Society: Towards a New Modernity*. London: Sage.

Blaxter, M. (1990). *Health and Lifestyles*. London: Sage.

Bruce, N. (1991) Epidemiology and the new public health: Implications for training. *Social Science and Medicine*, 32(1), 103-106.

Buckworth, J. and Dishman, R. (2002). *Exercise Psychology*. London. Human Kinetics.

Burke, V., Milligan, R.A., Beilin, L.J., Dunbar, D., Spencer, M., Balde, E. and Gracey, M.P. (1997). Clustering of health-related behaviours among 18 year old Australians. *Preventative Medicine*, 26, 724-733.

Center for Disease Control. (2007). *Healthy Youth! Sexual Risk Behaviours*. Avaliable at: http://www.cdc.gov/HealthyYouth/sexualbehaviors/index.htm (accessed 20 December 2007).

Craig, R. and Mindell, J. (2008). *Health Survey for England 2006. Volume 1: Cardiovascular Disease and Risk Factors in Adults*. London: The Information Centre.

Delaney, W.P. and Ames, G. (1995). Work team attitudes, drinking norms and workplace drinking. *Journal of Drug Issues*, 25, 275.

Department of Health. (1999). *Saving Lives: Our Healthier Nation*. London: The Stationery Office.

Department of Health. (2004). *At Least Five a Week: Evidence on the Impact of Physical Activity and its Relationship to Health*. London: Department of Health.

Doyle, R. (2001). Lifestyle blues. *Scientific American*, 284, 30.

Emslie, C., Hunt, K. and Macintyre, S. (2002). How similar are the smoking and drinking habits of men and women in non-manual jobs? *European Journal of Public Health*, 12, 22-28.

European Monitoring Centre for Drugs and Drug Addiction. http://www.emcdda.europa.eu (Accessed 2009).

Folkard, S., Lombardi, D.A. and Tucker, P.T. (2005). Shiftwork: safety, sleepiness and sleep. *Industrial Health*, 43, 20-23.

Fox, K.R. and Hillsdon, M. (2007). Physical activity and obesity. *Obesity Reviews*, 8(Suppl. 1), 115-121.

Gard, M. and Wright, J. (2005). *The Obesity Epidemic*. London: Routledge.

Hansen, E. and Easthope, G. (2007) *Lifestyle in Medicine*. London: Routledge.

Haslam, D. (2007). Obesity: A medical history. *Obesity Reviews*, 8(Suppl. 1), 31-36.

HM Government. (2007). *Safe. Sensible. Social. The Next Steps in the National Alcohol Strategy*. London: Department of Health and The Home Office.

Jeffery, R.W., Baxter, J.E., McGuire, M.T. and Linde, J.A. (2006). Are fast food restaurants an environmental risk factor for obesity? *International Journal of Behaviour, Nutrition and Physical Activity*, 3, 2.

Jones, A., Bentham, G., Foster, C., Hillsdon, M. and Panter, J. (2007). *Tackling Obesities: Future Choices – Obesogenic Environments – Evidence Review*. London: United Kingdom Government Foresight Programme, Office of Science and Innovation. Crown Copyright.

McPearson, P.D. (1992). Health for all Australians. In H. Gardner (ed) *Health Policy*. Melbourne: Churchhill Livingstone.

Myslobodsky, M. (2003) Gorurmand savants and environmental determinants of obesity. *Obesity Reviews*, 4, 121–128.

Nielsen, S.J. and Popkin, B.M. (2003) Patterns and trends in food portion sizes, 1977–1998. *Journal of the American Medical Association*, 289, 450–453.

Nursing Times (accessed 2009). www.nursingtimes.net

Office for National Statistics. (ONS). (2007). *Social Trends*, 2007. Newport: ONS.

Plant, M. and Plant, M. (2006). *Binge Britain*. Oxford: Oxford University Press.

Scambler, G. (ed) (2003). *Sociology as Applied to Medicine*, 5th edn. London: Elsevier.

Schubotz, D., Simpson, A. and Rolston, B. (2003). Towards better sexual health: A survey of sexual attitudes and lifestyles of young people in Northern Ireland. Research Report. Belfast: fpa in partnership with the University of Ulster.

Scotland Health Improvement Agency. Health Improvement Agency. http://www.healthscotland.com/ (accessed 23 November 2009).

Thirlaway, K.J. and Heggs, D. (2005). Interpreting risk messages: Women's responses to a health story. *Health, Risk and Society*, 7, 107–121.

Thomas, R. (1811) *The Modern Practice of Physic*. New York: Collins and Co.

Townsend, P. and Davidson, N. (1989) *Inequalities in Health: The Black Report*. Harmondsworth: Penguin.

Wardle, J. and Steptoe, A. (2005) Public health psychology. *The Psychologist*, 18, 672–675.

Welsh Assembly Government (accessed 2009). http://new.wales.gov.uk/topics/health/improvement/healthatwork/corporate-standard/?lang=en

Wiseman, M. (2009). www.wcrf-uk.org

World Health Organisation (Health Education Unit). (1986). Lifestyles and health. *Social Science in Medicine*, 22, 117–124.

Chapter 2
Psychology in practice

LEARNING OBJECTIVES

At the end of this chapter you will:

- Have been introduced to the key psychological factors that influence behavioural change
- Recognise the key barriers to behavioural change
- Have evaluated how psychological approaches can improve the likelihood of clients following behavioural advice
- Recognise that getting people to adopt a healthy behaviour is only the start of a process and that people will need continued support to maintain a change
- Have considered the unique problems involved with attempting to change well-established habits

Case study

Caroline is a practice nurse in a semi-urban GP practice. Her role at the clinic includes health promotion. When Caroline first joined the practice she was very enthusiastic about the health promotion aspect of her role. She was convinced of the importance of a healthy lifestyle in preventing chronic disease. Caroline set up a high blood pressure clinic and a weight control clinic to support patients who had been advised by the doctor to reduce their blood pressure and/or lose weight. Caroline sees patients shortly after the doctor has told them that they are putting their health at risk; many are worried and anxious about their future health. Patients at these clinics are provided with high-quality information and advice about how to change their diet, reduce their drinking and increase their physical activity. They are directed towards local leisure-centre classes and given suggested meal plans. However, over the five years that Caroline has worked at the practice she has become disillusioned with her health promotion role. Very few people make permanent changes to their eating, drinking or exercise habits and the number of patients diagnosed with type 2 diabetes and other chronic diseases continues to increase.

At first, Caroline wondered whether her patients didn't understand the health information that she was giving them. However, a questionnaire survey amongst the clinic attendees demonstrated that the majority understood the importance of a healthy lifestyle, were aware of the government recommendations for diet and exercise and knew about the local community leisure facilities. Caroline has come to the conclusion that education is not going to result in lots of patients changing their ways and is looking for new approaches to use in her clinic. She has enrolled on a continuing professional development (CPD) module looking at psychological approaches to behavioural change in the hope that it will give her new ideas improve her practice.

Discussion point

Consider the reasons why Caroline's clients do not follow her advice.

Introduction

The central strategy of health promotion has always been education. Health education involves a combination of risk communication and behavioural advice. As such, it assumes that people practise unhealthy lifestyle behaviours because they do not understand what is bad or good for their health and that if they had correct information they would make healthy choices.

In line with an educational approach to health promotion, until recently psychology has focused on investigating how people understand and respond to the information they receive about health and behaviour. This is often described as a social cognitive approach to behavioural change. Social cognitive approaches assume that behavioural choices are a reflection of the way people see and think about the world. Consequently, if we can understand how people think then we will be able to influence the way they decide to behave. A key aspect of this approach is the recognition that different people may perceive the same thing differently. So what is unpleasant for one person may be enjoyable for another. In terms of lifestyle choices, one person may find cycling to work a pleasant way to unwind after work, whilst another cannot face cycling home at the end of a long day.

Decisions about how to behave are thought to involve some sort of cost-benefit analysis. In its simplest version, any model of behavioural change is a straightforward weighing up of these two factors (Figure 2.1). Research has then gone on to investigate what other factors are also influential. A number of different theoretical models of health behaviour have been developed to predict people's behavioural choices, all expansions of the basic cost-benefit model (Figure 2.1). It is beyond the remit of this text to provide a description and explanation of the numerous social cognitive models of behaviour. There are a number of texts where the reader can find a comprehensive review of these models, such as Conner and Norman (2005) or Thirlaway and Upton (2009). In this chapter we will evaluate the key factors (Table 2.1) that emerge from research on the various social cognitive models of behaviour as particularly influential on behavioural change.

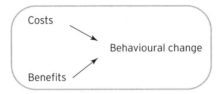

Figure 2.1 A cost-benefit model of behavioural change

What, in your experience, do you think are important factors in the decision to change behaviour?

Promoting lifestyle change has traditionally focused on educating people to realise that they need to change and more recently on motivating people so that they wish to change. However, the focus on getting people to adopt healthier habits has been at the expense of considering how people maintain newly adopted habits (Nigg et al., 2008). Lifestyle change needs to be long term to improve health outcomes but unfortunately many people who take up a healthy behaviour soon stop. For example, research has shown that about 50% of people who start a formal physical activity programme drop out within six months (Nigg et al., 2008). Psychological concepts such as self-regulation, habituation and stages of change do recognise the long-term issues around behavioural change and the interventions associated with these concepts go some way towards addressing the issue of sustained change (Table 2.1).

Table 2.1 Factors that may influence lifestyle behavioural change

Psychological concept	Associated intervention
Perception of risk	Education
Perception of benefits	Education
Barriers	Structural change
Social norms	Policy; education; cultural adaptation
Social support	Motivational interviewing; counselling
Self-efficacy	Motivational interviewing; goal setting
Self-regulation	Goal setting; implementation intentions
Fear	Risk communication
Habituation	Motivational interviewing; implementation intentions; cognitive behavioural therapy
Pleasure	Little known, classical conditioning
Stages of change	Various, depending on stage

Psychological concepts

Perception of risk and benefits

A perception of risk is a central factor in the majority of psychological models of behavioural change; it delivers the costs side of the basic behavioural change evaluation (Figure 2.1). It is assumed that unless people realise that a behaviour is risky they will not attempt to alter that behaviour.

In 2002 the Cabinet Office Strategy Unit defined risk as:

Uncertainty of outcome, whether positive opportunity or negative threat.
(Cabinet Office Strategy Unit, 2002, p. 7)

However, for most people risk is negative and indicates something to worry about (Thirlaway and Heggs, 2005). Indeed, a lot of risk communication is intended to generate fear and anxiety in order to get people to change their behaviour; whether this works will be considered later in the chapter.

A more useful definition of risk for health promotion is the one provided by Connolly *et al.* (2000):

A situation of risk presents some chance of injury, damage or loss, a hazard or dangerous chance.

So the starting point for any health promotion activity has always been to communicate a risk because it is assumed that unless people realise that drinking is dangerous they are unlikely to stop (Photograph 2.1). Similarly, people are unlikely to adopt healthy behaviours that they don't enjoy, such as eating fruit, unless they understand that not eating fruit puts their health at risk.

Health professionals collectively make a decision about what is risky and what is safe. They provide a plethora of information about the 'right' way to behave. In the UK people are advised about the number of units of alcohol they can safely consume. They are advised to eat five portions of fruit and vegetables each day and to do 30 minutes of moderate to vigorous physical activity each week. There is expert advice available on the correct way to brush

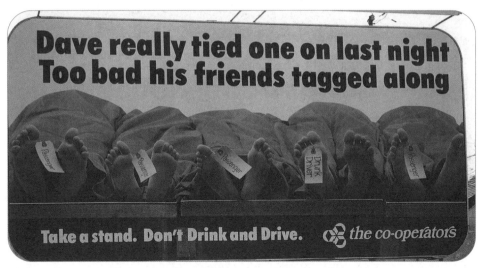

Photograph 2.1 Risk communication about the dangers of drink-driving
Source: The Advertising Archives

your teeth, the amount of water to drink, the speed at which to drive your car. Through risk communication the government informs us both of the *cost* of practising unhealthy behaviours, such as drinking too much, and of the *cost* of avoiding healthy behaviours, such as being physically active. There is an agreed 'correct' risk perception and on the basis of that, an agreed 'correct' decision. However, health promotion has been communicating lifestyle risks for more than two decades with little impact on lifestyle choices. In general the public fail to adhere to the recommendations made by the government (Department of Health, 1999). It is often assumed that this is because they don't understand the risk correctly (Thirlaway and Upton, 2009). Indeed, in 1999 the Department of Health stated that lay risk perceptions must be challenged by more effective risk communications. However, a large body of research suggests that people understand the risks associated with an unhealthy lifestyle perfectly well but still do not change their behaviour (Blaxter, 1990; Lawton and Conner, 2007).

Applying this to Caroline

Caroline needs to recognise that providing risk information is only a small aspect of the behavioural change intervention process.

The other main communication that health promotion delivers is behavioural advice and this behavioural advice often informs about the *benefits* of change (Photograph 2.2) as well giving advice about what the change should be. Similarly to risk communications, behavioural advice is generally well understood but it is not generally adhered to (Thirlaway and Upton, 2009).

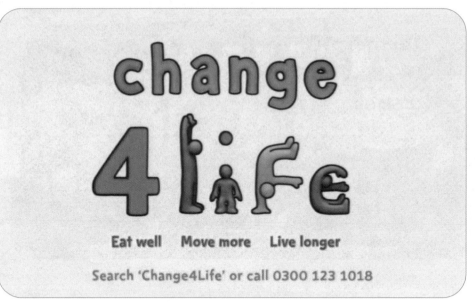

Photograph 2.2 Benefits communication
Source: The Advertising Archives

Applying this to Caroline

Once Caroline has recognised that educating people about the risks (costs) of unhealthy behaviour and the benefits of healthy behaviour will not, on its own, result in behavioural change, she will need to explore what other strategies she can use to improve the uptake of and adherence to the advice she provides.

Why don't people respond to risk communications and behavioural advice about their lifestyle by changing their behaviour? Certainly, when asked to evaluate a risky communication people report feeling anxious or worried (Thirlaway and Heggs, 2005). It has been argued by Thirlaway and Upton (2009) that there are three main reasons why risk communications do not result in lifestyle behavioural change.

Firstly, lifestyle behaviours are not practised solely for health reasons. Lifestyle behaviours have other social outcomes that are often more important for people than a future risk to health, so any cost-benefit analysis carried out by individuals may include non-health outcomes that are often not considered by health-focused health professionals.

Secondly, health messages are predominantly focused on long-term health outcomes. This requires people to be 'future-orientated' and most people are focused in the present (Thirlaway and Upton, 2009). Health promotion is asking people to make unpalatable changes to their life now in order to reduce a risk that is a long way in the future. Consequently, people tend to look for other, less difficult ways to reduce the anxiety that a risk communication generates. It is easier to use strategies such as deciding the source of the message is untrustworthy, or to be unrealistically optimistic about your current behaviour, than it is to actually set about changing.

Thirdly, many established health behaviours have become habitual and are controlled not by cognitive decisions but by automatic responses to the routine situations of our daily lives (Aarts *et al.*, 1997). How many of us have decided to give up biscuits with our cup of coffee only to find that we are halfway through one before we remember our decision not to eat them?

Key message

Getting people to change their lifestyle requires them to make unpalatable changes in the present for an uncertain benefit in the future. It requires them to prioritise their health and to attempt to break often well-established habits.

Barriers

Barriers refer to those things that are part of our wider social and physical environment that prevent us carrying out behaviours we might otherwise choose to do. Individuals tend to list a set of barriers, such as lack of time, lack of resources, or poor facilities, as the reason for their failure to make positive lifestyle choices. However, what is a barrier for one person, e.g. a three-mile trip to a leisure centre, may not be seen as a barrier at all for another.

Key message

It is the way people perceive their social and physical environment rather than their actual environment that is important.

The term obesogenic environment is now widely used to refer to the physical, economic, social and cultural barriers in the environment that impede the maintenance of a healthy body weight (Swinburn *et al.*, 1999). Barriers to successful weight maintenance are things like the easy availability of high-fat food and the environmental obstacles to active commuting. However, recently the government-commissioned Foresight Report on obesity in the UK (Jones *et al.*, 2007) concluded that the influence of the environment on obesity was not straightforward. It is not the environment *per se* that matters but the way individuals perceive it. Jones *et al.*, (2007) and Mutrie *et al.* (2002) have raised concerns that building more cycle paths may only encourage people who already cycle rather than creating more cyclists. They both argue that non-cyclists will need support to encourage them to believe that they could use the cycle paths provided in their environment.

Discussion point

How could Caroline go about changing her clients' perceptions of the local resources available to them to increase their physical activity?

Social norms

As part of their detailed analysis of obesity in the UK the Foresight authors (Jones *et al.*, 2007) argue that normative social behaviour, that is, what is acceptable behaviour to the majority of an individual's peer group, is key to understanding and promoting positive lifestyle choices (Jones *et al.*, 2007). For a number of decades psychologists have found very little evidence that social norms are influential over lifestyle choices but it appears that they may have been asking the wrong questions (Thirlaway and Upton, 2009). Psychologists have carried out a lot of research looking at what is socially acceptable or unacceptable, and how motivated people are to comply with what is expected of them. Looked at in this way, there is very little evidence that social norms influence behaviour (Godin and Kok, 1996). However, more recently, in the field of drinking research has focused on looking at how much individuals think their peers are drinking (Kuther and Timoshin, 2003). This is a much more promising line of research and there is a clear relationship between what people think their peers are drinking and what they themselves choose to drink. This relationship has been demonstrated both in adults at work and in students at college (Kuther and Timoshin, 2003; Barrientos-Gutierrez et al., 2007). The fact that people are influenced in their drinking by what they think other people are drinking is particularly interesting because of the wealth of evidence that indicates people are generally very optimistic about their own behaviour in comparison to other people (Weinstein, 1984).

Applying this to Caroline

Caroline could use data from individuals similar to her clients to demonstrate that their behaviour is actually more risky than that of other similar people.

Social support

There is considerable evidence that social isolation or lack of social support increases the risk of developing a range of chronic diseases (Wang *et al.*, 2005). Social support clearly matters for health but what is difficult is defining and measuring something so complex. As social support is fundamentally about relationships, a simple way to investigate social support is to count how many relationships an individual has. Other studies have tried to evaluate the quality of social support using questionnaires that ask questions such as:

Do you have someone that you can share your innermost thoughts with and confide in?
(Wang *et al.*, 2005, p. 600)

Another way to think about social support is in terms of emotional support (availability of close emotional support) and social integration (availability of peripheral contacts). Social support is a complex thing; we know that it has health benefits but it is hard to identify how it is beneficial and therefore develop any strategies to build in what is lacking for the socially isolated.

One way that social support is believed to improve health is by enhancing healthy lifestyles. For example, smokers with good social support are more likely to succeed in giving up smoking (Pirie *et al.*, 1997). Jeffery and French (1996) found that social class was related to obesity in women. One difference between women from different socio-economic groups is the perceived social support from friends for healthy diet and exercise behaviours, with women from higher social classes perceiving friends as more supportive.

What is not clear is whether general social support (good emotional support and/or strong social integration) is enough to support individuals attempting to change their behaviour or whether specific support for the attempted activity is necessary. So is it enough to get general emotional support from a partner whilst dieting, or does the partner need to be supportive of the specific dieting behaviour? Similarly, it is not clear whether specific support for changing behaviour, such as that available from personal trainers or support groups, is sufficient to support long-term behavioural change and could provide the social support necessary to facilitate change for the socially isolated. It has been argued that general social support improves health outcomes by acting as a stress buffer (Wang *et al.*, 2005). Individuals who have people with whom they can talk through stressful situations and from whom they can receive emotional support may receive direct physiological benefits in terms of lower levels of stress hormones (Wang *et al.*, 2005). Equally, they may be less likely to use alcohol, high-fat food or drugs as a stress alleviator (Gruber, 2008). Specific social support such as that provided by weight reduction groups, exercise programme classes or by personal trainers or other health professionals can work at the individual level by providing positive feedback about successful behavioural change and improving self-efficacy (Gruber, 2008) but it can also, over time, provide some of the general emotional support if the relationships persist over time.

Applying this to Caroline

Caroline needs to tailor her advice to ensure it does not threaten valuable social networks and increase stress for her clients.

Self-Efficacy

Self-efficacy is the belief that you can carry out a specific behaviour in a specific situation (Bandura, 1997). Self-efficacy has been found to be the best predictor of whether people will change their behaviour across all lifestyle behaviours. University students who reported higher levels of exercise self-efficacy were more likely to be physically active (Rovnaik *et al.*, 2002). Kuther and Timoshin (2003) found that those who believed they could control their drinking drank less. Higher self-efficacy has been found to predict greater ability to resist peer pressure to have sex (Dilorio *et al.*, 2001) and a better ability to avoid risky sexual behaviour (Faryna and Morales, 2000).

Key message

Individuals may understand the risks of continuing an unhealthy behaviour and the benefits of adopting a healthy behaviour, but unless they believe that they are capable of change they are unlikely to succeed in changing.

Self-efficacy is behaviour specific and is not transferable. So you may have high self-efficacy for taking physical activity but low self-efficacy for practising safe sex. Increasing self-efficacy in one behaviour will not translate into increased self-efficacy in other behaviours. Given the importance of self-efficacy in behavioural change, it is crucial to understand how self-efficacy can be improved or damaged.

The dieting industry is often detrimental to the self-efficacy of individuals trying to lose weight. There are many diets on the market offering rapid weight loss that is either very difficult to achieve or very difficult to maintain. A series of failed dieting attempts can seriously damage self-efficacy for weight loss. Professionals working with individuals trying to lose weight need to be aware that if they have made multiple failed attempts to lose weight and/or maintain weight loss they are likely to have very little confidence in their ability to succeed. Repeated failure is very damaging to self-efficacy.

Self-efficacy has been argued to be enhanced by personal accomplishment, mastery, vicarious experience or verbal persuasion (Walker, 2001). The strong evidence that increasing self-efficacy can promote behavioural change has generated a number of psychological strategies to support self-efficacy, including motivational interviewing, goal setting and implementation intentions, all of which will be discussed later in the chapter.

Applying this to Caroline

Caroline may want to consider how confident her clinic participants are about making the changes she is suggesting and investigate ways of increasing their self-efficacy for the proposed change.

Self-regulation

Self-regulation in the context of behavioural change refers to efforts by people to alter their responses to situational cues such as being in a pub and not ordering an alcoholic drink. It is people trying to control the number of calories they consume, the number of units of alcohol they drink, the drugs they take, the cigarettes they consume, the time they spend in sedentary activities or the amount of physical activity they take. It is likely that at any one time a majority of people will be attempting to regulate one or more of their lifestyle behaviours. The chronic diseases that are the major health issues for people in the twenty-first century can all be argued to be influenced by people's failure to control their appetites for pleasure-giving substances or behaviours. Self-regulation is closely linked to self-efficacy because if people try and succeed in regulating a behaviour their self-efficacy will increase. However, if they try and fail to regulate a behaviour they risk damaging their self-efficacy and are less likely to succeed if they attempt regulation again.

Successful self-regulation involves setting goals for a particular behaviour and sticking to them. So, for instance, many people try to lose weight by going on a calorie-controlled diet where they attempt to limit the amount of calories they consume each day. Interestingly, people who are dieting are more prone to bouts of disinhibited eating than people who are not attempting to diet. At first sight this is counterintuitive, in that people who are trying to restrict their calorie intake should be less likely to overeat. However, research consistently shows that if people on a diet are asked to consume food perceived as 'high calorie', such as a rich milkshake, they are more likely than people not dieting to over-consume afterwards when provided with palatable food (Herman and Polivy, 2004). It would seem that once dieters perceive that they have 'failed' to stick to their daily calorie quota, they feel they might as well eat whatever they like. Herman and Polivy (2004, p.498) describe this as the 'what-the-hell' effect. This then creates a real problem for health professionals attempting to encourage weight loss because the setting of goals for calorie intake may actually put individuals at greater risk of overeating. In the field of alcohol and drug addiction many treatment programmes aim for total abstinence, which is one response to the problem of disinhibition; however, total abstinence is not an option for sustained weight loss.

Key message

Self-regulation requires the setting of goals but failing to achieve goals appears to put people at greater risk of excessive consumption and/or damaged self-efficacy.

Fear

When the relationship between behaviour and health was first recognised and health professionals wanted to stop unhealthy behaviours they used risk communication to try to generate fear (Photograph 2.3).

Fear appeals are based on the fear-drive model which argues that fear is unpleasant and people want to avoid it. If a communication makes people feel fearful or anxious, as the advertisement in Photograph 2.3 is intended to do, then the fear-drive model suggests that the recipient will want to reduce this unpleasant state of mind. If the communication also

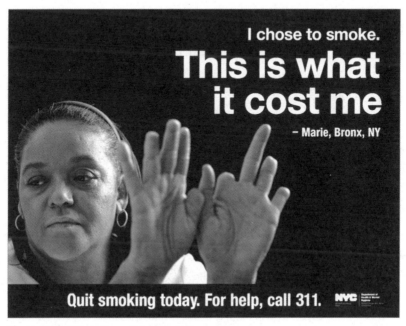

Photograph 2.3 Anti-smoking advertisement
Source: © DOHMH

contains advice, like the advertisement in Photograph 2.3, then individuals may try to follow this advice in order to escape from the unpleasant feelings of anxiety and fear for their future health. If following the behavioural advice leads to a reduction in fear then people are likely to continue with their changed behaviour.

Fear is intuitively appealing as a means of promoting behavioural change but the role it plays in initiating behavioural change is not clear-cut or consistent (Janis, 1968; Nabi, 2002; Bandura, 1998). Rigby *et al.* (1989) reported that the Australian 'Grim Reaper' campaign raised anxiety and awareness of HIV and AIDS but failed to increase knowledge or facilitate a change in behaviour.

Often the response to failed fear appeals is to increase the level of fear either by increasing the graphicness of the imagery or by focusing on the worst possible outcome. Photograph 2.4 is an example of a risk communication about smoking that is both more graphic than the communication in Photograph 2.3 and focuses on the fatal consequences of smoking rather than the disfigurement portrayed in Photograph 2.4.

However, the evidence suggests that increasing the level of fear generated by a message does not increase the uptake of behavioural prevention strategies. One reason may be that highly fearful messages are likely to induce denial and therefore fail to have any impact on behavioural choices (Sutton, 1982).

Key message

It seems logical to assume that anxious and worried people will follow advice that will reduce their risk but actually fear is not a good motivator of behavioural change.

Habituation

Past behaviour is a powerful predictor of future behaviour (Hagger *et al.*, 2002; Conner and Norman, 2005). Consistent patterns of past behaviours are often referred to as habits. Habits are behaviours that may once have been initiated by rational choice but are now

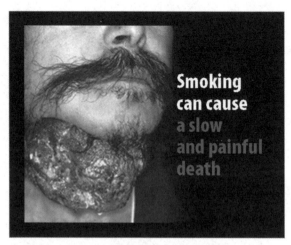

Photograph 2.4 A graphic image of the costs of smoking, with a clear message that smoking kills
Source: © European Union, 2010

under the control of specific situational cues that trigger the behaviour without thinking (Aarts *et al.*, 1997). So, many of the choices we make about what to eat for breakfast, the amount of coffee we consume, whether we walk or drive to work on a day-to-day basis are not conscious choices at all but things we do without thinking. Health promotion and social cognition, when looking at lifestyle behavioural change, assume that lifestyle choices are always a conscious choice, which may explain why their educational strategies are less effective than they would like.

All lifestyle behaviours have the potential to become habits or even addictions. There is a tendency to assume that behaviours such as smoking and drinking that include a physiological response to the alcohol or the nicotine are harder habits to break because of the combined physiological and psychological reinforcement. However, people struggle to give up smoking long after the physiological addiction is overcome (Thirlaway and Upton, 2009), which implies that psychological addiction can be powerful alone.

Key message

Lifestyle behaviours have the potential to be habitual or addictive, which means that even if people want to change and think they should change, they are going to find it difficult not to revert to their bad habits.

Health professionals are faced with a dual problem: they need to help people break unhealthy habits and they need to support the development of healthy habits. Many of the unhealthy habits that older adults struggle with, as the negative consequences of decades of unhealthy living start to materialise, are established in adolescence and early adulthood when health is optimal, and the costs of smoking, drinking, eating badly or not exercising are in the distant future. Important outcomes for young people are identity formation and the establishment of social relationships (Kuther and Timoshin, 2003). Drinking and eating are an integral component of many social events in the UK and alcohol in particular enhances social integration and facilitates the development of relationships. Interventions that attempt to enable young people to set up healthy drinking habits need to focus on the role of alcohol for young people in the present, rather than on the cost of alcohol consumption in the future. On a positive front, sport is often central to socialisation, particularly for young men, and supports the establishment of positive physical activity habits (Thirlaway and Upton, 2009).

Health starts to become pertinent for individuals as they start to experience ill-health and the costs of unhealthy lifestyles are in the present or the near future rather than in the distant future (Lawton, 2002). Unfortunately, by the time individuals wish to change their unhealthy habits they are likely to be well established and difficult to break. Research now needs to focus on understanding how we can help people change ingrained habits, and implementation intentions are one promising avenue.

Applying this to Caroline

Caroline needs to recognise that her clients are not disregarding her advice and probably leave her clinic with every intention to change but find it impossible to overcome ingrained habits.

Pleasure

People usually choose to do things that they enjoy. Pleasure can be argued to be the main motivation for lifestyle choices, particularly among the young (Orford, 2001). Pleasure can be experienced as a physiological sensation, for instance the response to chocolate in the mouth. Pleasure can also be experienced as a positive emotion, for instance winning a game of sport. Frequently, a pleasurable response includes both physiological and emotive sensations. Some things are innately pleasurable, such as sweet food. Other things we learn to enjoy, such as drinking alcohol. Few young people enjoy their first taste of an alcoholic drink, which is why beverage manufacturers have developed sweetened alcoholic drinks for the teenage market to make the alcohol more palatable and support the initiation of learnt enjoyment of alcohol (Plant and Plant, 2006).

Regardless of whether the pleasure is physiological or psychological, innate or learnt, if an experience is pleasurable people are more likely to repeat it. Consequently, pleasure is fundamental in the establishment of habitual behaviours. One approach to encouraging healthy lifestyle habits would be to try to elicit pleasurable responses to healthy behaviours. However, we don't understand very well how people learn to enjoy certain behaviours and not others.

Applying this to Caroline

Presumably most health professionals understand that people do things that they enjoy but they seldom take that into account when offering advice about lifestyle change.

Stages of change

As well as looking at what external factors influence behavioural change, psychologists have also looked at the motivation state of the individual who is trying to change. This approach views change not as a one-off event but as a process, and argues that health professionals need to tailor their support for individuals to their stage of change.

According to all stage theories, a person can move through a series of stages in the process of behavioural change. Different models argue for different numbers of stages that last for differing lengths of time. The most well-known stages of change model comes from the transtheoretical model of change which conceptualises the process of change as having five stages as described in Table 2.2.

The model argues that it is important to understand where people are in the process of change before attempting to support them to change, because depending on the stage of change you would use different techniques to encourage a change in behaviour. For example, if people are in the pre-contemplation stage you may use education to move them into contemplation. Once people are contemplating a change then motivational interviewing may be key to encouraging people to start preparing to change. During the stages of preparation and action, strategies to increase self-efficacy may be important. Which interventions are best at different stages is not well established (Thirlaway and Upton, 2009).

Table 2.2 The stages of change, conceptualised using alcohol as the health behaviour

Stages of change	Behavioural and motivational characteristics
Pre-contemplation	Individuals are drinking and have no intention of stopping in the next six months
Contemplation	Individuals are drinking but they intend to stop in the next six months
Preparation	Individuals are drinking less and intend to stop in the next six months
Action	Individuals have stopped drinking to excess within the past six months. The perceived benefits are greater than the perceived costs. This is the least stable stage
Maintenance	Individuals have been non-drinkers for over six months and risk of relapse is small

Applying this to Caroline

Caroline could consider tailoring her approach so that she focused on providing behavioural advice to those clients who are contemplating or preparing to change.

Psychological interventions

Motivational interviewing

Miller and Rollnick (2002) suggested that motivation is fundamental to change and they suggest that motivational interviewing is the appropriate approach. Motivational interviewing can be defined as 'a client-centred, directive method for enhancing intrinsic motivation to change by exploring and resolving ambivalence' (Miller and Rollnick, 2002).

Key message

The aim of motivational interviewing is to increase an individual's motivation to change.

Motivational interviewing aims to increase an individual's motivation to consider change rather than showing them how to change. If a person doesn't want to change then it is irrelevant if they know how to do it or not. However, if a person is motivated to change then the interventions aimed at changing behaviour can begin.

Motivational interviewing (MI) is a technique based on cognitive-behavioural therapy which aims to enhance an individual's motivation to change health behaviour. The whole process aims to help the patient understand their thought processes, to identify how their thought processes are helping to produce the inappropriate behaviour and how their thought processes can be changed to develop alternative, health-promoting, behaviours. Motivational interviewing differs from counselling because it is directive; the healthcare professional elicits and selectively reinforces change talk that resolves ambivalence and moves the client towards change.

Motivational strategies include eight components that are designed to increase the level of motivation the person has towards changing a specific behaviour. It is important to note that the motivation is specific to one behaviour and so being motivated to quit smoking does not simply transfer to being motivated to reduce alcohol consumption. The eight components are:

- giving advice (about specific behaviours to be changed);
- removing barriers (often about access to particular help);
- providing choice (making it clear that if they choose not to change that is their right and it is their choice; the therapist is there to encourage change but not to insist on change);
- decreasing desirability (of the ambivalence towards change or the status quo);
- practising empathy;
- providing feedback (from a variety of perspectives – family, friends, health professionals – in order to give the patient a full picture of their current situation);
- clarifying goals (feedback should be compared with a standard (an ideal), and clarification of the ideal can provide the pathway to the goal);
- active helping (such as expressing caring or facilitating a referral, both of which convey a real interest in helping the person to change).

Although this seems relatively simple and straightforward and, to a certain extent, it is, there are a number of key skills that you need to employ in order to be successful in motivating people to change and some of these are presented in Table 2.3.

Goal setting

We all set ourselves goals in all areas of life. Some psychologists would argue that goals give meaning to people's lives (Rasmussen *et al.*, 2006). The challenge for health professionals interested in behavioural change is how to utilise goal setting to support change. Goals can vary both in terms of their difficulty (running a marathon is more difficult that running a 10 km race) and in terms of their specificity (Strecher *et al.*, 1995). Someone may have a vague goal 'to eat well' or a more specific goal 'to eat a high-fibre breakfast cereal at least five times a week'.

Evidence suggests that non-specific, vague goals such as wanting to lose weight are less likely to be achieved than more specific goals such as 'I am going to stop eating chocolate biscuits for the next fortnight' (Strecher *et al.*, 1995). Health professionals therefore can support people in their overarching goals to lose weight, get fitter, control their blood sugar etc. by helping them break down down their complex and long-term goals into a set of simpler, short-term sub-goals.

A major benefit of goal-directed behaviour is the possibility of positive feedback. Feedback about goal success can significantly improve subsequent performance, probably by improving self-efficacy. However, for behavioural change, difficult, complex, long-term goals

Table 2.3 Key skills for motivational interviewing

Skill	Comment
Express empathy	There should be no criticism or blame as acceptance facilitates change
Develop discrepancy	Change is motivated by a perceived discrepancy between present behaviour and personal goal
Roll with resistance	Avoid arguing for change or providing change – see the smoker as the source of information
Support self-efficacy	The smoker's belief in the possibility of change is an important motivator for change
Use open-ended questions	Encourage the client to do most of the talking: 'What are your concerns about smoking?'
Use reflective listening	Reflect back change talk in a statement: 'I had real cravings this morning' to 'You are a little concerned about the cravings in the morning'
Use affirmation	Use to build rapport: 'You are right to be concerned about smoking in front of the children'
Summarise	Link together and reinforce what has been discussed: 'You are concerned that your smoking may cause lung cancer'
Reframe or agree with a twist	Address resistance by reinterpreting: 'My kids nag me about giving up smoking' to 'It sounds like they really care about your health'
Emphasise personal choice	Reinforce that it is the client's choice to change their behaviour
Evocative questions	
Increasing confidence	Use open questions to evoke confidence talk: 'How might you go about making this change?'
Confidence ruler	Use the ruler to ask 'What would it take to score higher?'
Strengths and successes	Review obstacles and how the client has overcome them
Reframing	'I've tried three times to quit and failed' to 'You have had three good attempts already and are learning new skills'
Prompt coping strategies	Ask for potential obstacles and putative coping strategies

Source: Adapted from Miller and Rollnick (2002)

(such as weight loss or fitness) are unlikely to generate immediate positive feedback. This can lead to a reduction in self-efficacy as individuals feel they are not achieving their goal and can lead to individuals giving up and reverting to their original 'bad habits'. Indeed, research suggests that failing to achieve self-regulatory goals can promote a worsening of original bad habits (Herman and Polivy, 2004). Short-term goals are much easier to link to positive feedback and can improve self-efficacy and help people stick to their change. The majority of health behaviours that people wish to change are highly complex and will require careful planning to develop an appropriate goal-setting strategy. It is generally better to set behavioural goals such as increasing exercise rather than physiological status goals such as increasing VO2 max. Behaviours are more directly under a person's control than are physiological responses. The key strategies for successful goal setting are presented in Table 2.4.

It is emerging that having an action plan about how to achieve goals that involve particularly ingrained habitual behaviours can be further supported by 'if-then' plans that provide strategies for people to achieve their goals in difficult contexts (see following section on implementation intentions).

Successful goal setting will promote self-efficacy for changing the specified behaviour, giving the client the confidence to believe that having met previous goals, they can meet the next sub-goal and that the overarching goal is possible. Ineffective goal setting, when clients fail to meet their short-term targets, can have the opposite effect and damage self-efficacy, reducing the likelihood that clients will meet their overarching goal.

Effective goal setting needs to be tailored to the individual and supported by regular feedback and encouragement. For long-term goals, such as major weight loss, this will involve considerable and sustained input from a health professional. It is not usual for health professionals to have the resources available to provide this level of individualised support. One avenue that might be worthy of exploration is whether clients can be taught effective goal-setting techniques and could then set and reward their own goals.

Table 2.4   Key recommendations for goal-setting behavioural change strategies using weight loss as the example

Strategy	Example
Explore client motivation. This might be done using the stages of change paradigm. Pre-contemplation clients are not ready for goal setting	A client has been referred to you by her GP for weight loss support. The client has been advised to lose 3 stone. Initially, you need to establish the client's personal motivation for weight loss of this magnitude
Break down a complex goal into a series of short-term sub-goals and create an action plan	You might set the client a series of short-term goals such as stop eating biscuits at coffee time for the next fortnight
Attempt where possible to set behavioural goals rather than physiological goals	You may wish to focus on the food an individual chooses to eat or on an activity such as walking rather than pounds lost over a time frame
Evaluate client self-efficacy for the various behaviours involved in goal achievement	Your client may be more confident about restricting food intake than taking exercise and your action plan needs to be tailored to client self-efficacy
Tailor sub-goals to the client to ensure they are challenging but realistic and perceived as such by the client	Your client may wish to set goals that are unrealistic, as rapid weight loss is attractive to most individuals wishing to lose weight. You need to negotiate a goal for which you are likely to be able to deliver positive feedback
Provide regular feedback to the client	Feedback needs to be regular, supportive and reflect behavioural achievements and physiological achievements if appropriate
Goal adaptation	For long-term complex change the short-term sub-goals may need to be reviewed and renegotiated as the client's physiological status and self-efficacy change in response to behavioural adaptation

> ## Key message
>
> Effective self-regulation requires the setting of challenging but realistic short-term goals that support the development of self-efficacy.

Implementation intentions

One of the problems with goal setting and with behavioural change generally is that people may have decided to change, they may want to change very strongly, but because their behaviour is habitual and ingrained they may not be able to overcome the impulse to give in, in situations where they habitually practise an unhealthy behaviour. So people who are trying to give up smoking will have key situational prompts when they find it very hard to overcome the impulse to smoke; perhaps during a coffee break, or in the pub. Gollwitzer and Sheeran (2006) have suggested that people need to develop a set of 'if-then' plans to help them deal with situations where they usually do something they are trying to stop doing. For example, if your goal is to lose weight then you need to identify when you are likely to eat high-fat food and how you will respond differently in that situation. So if you usually have a cup of tea and a biscuit mid-morning you need to formulate an alternative response to replace eating a biscuit, such as eating a low-fat cracker instead.

Building 'if-then' plans into goal-setting action plans increases the involvement and commitment of the health professional. As mentioned under goal setting, it is unlikely that many health professionals currently have the resources to provide this level of support. Research is urgently required to establish how effective such tailored individualised interventions could be, the minimum level of professional input necessary for success and the economic advantages of such potentially preventative interventions.

Cognitive behavioural therapy

Cognitive behavioural therapy (CBT) is more traditionally associated with mental health disorders (such as anxiety, depression, panic or agoraphobia) than with lifestyle choices (Westbrook *et al.*, 2007). However, CBT may well be useful for some individuals attempting to change their lifestyle. Indeed, motivational interviewing (described earlier in the chapter) is based on aspects of CBT. However, in some instances, perhaps when the behaviour people are attempting to change is clearly addictive, there may be a place for a more complete cognitive behavioural approach than motivational interviewing. Motivational interviewing is usually a brief therapy (1-4 sessions) for enhancing motivation to change problematic health behaviours (Ismail *et al.*, 2008). Cognitive behavioural therapy is longer (a minimum of six sessions) and aims to help the client identify, challenge and substitute unhelpful thoughts (cognitions) and behaviours with more constructive ones (Ismail *et al.*, 2008). It is beyond the remit of this book to provide a comprehensive review of CBT and the reader is advised to access one of the many available texts if they wish to explore the subject further (for instance: Westbrook *et al.*, 2007). Ismail *et al.* (2008) found that CBT improved blood glucose control in patients with diabetes 12 months after the intervention whereas motivational interviewing did not. However, given that motivational interviewing is a brief intervention and CBT is a longer-term intervention, it is possible that it is the length of the intervention that results in the better outcome rather than the type of therapy itself. Longer-term interventions have the potential to provide social support for individuals attempting to change a behaviour, and it may be the social support rather than the therapeutic approach that is important.

Conclusion

The various behaviours implicated in contributing to ill-health – eating, drinking, smoking, illicit drug taking and sexual behaviours – are all complex behaviours that have many different roles in individuals' lives. People need to eat to stay alive and hunger is the physiological response that ensures that people do eat and don't starve to death. Viewed in this simplistic way, understanding eating behaviour should be straightforward. People should eat enough to prevent hunger. However, people eat for pleasure, they eat for comfort, they eat because they are bored, they eat because the social situation demands it, they eat because they have got into the habit of doing so in particular situations or at particular times. Psychological theories of behavioural change have developed to try to understand how these non-biological factors influence the choices people make. Psychological theory to date gives us some clues about the key factors that influence behaviour.

Putting this into action

- Don't think the job is done once people understand the risk. Risk information will not promote behavioural change in the majority of people.
- Try to understand how the behaviours you are trying to change are involved in an individual's social networks. How much social support will be available for the proposed change?
- Evaluate an individual's readiness for change and tailor the intervention to their motivational state.
- Evaluate an individual's self-efficacy and set goals that will increase self-efficacy.
- Recognise where there are habitual patterns of behaviour and develop implementation strategies to overcome the compulsion to revert to old habits.

Summary Points

- Education about the risks and benefits of behaviour is not an effective behavioural change strategy.
- Getting people to change their lifestyle requires them to prioritise their health and change often long-established habits.
- Getting people to change their lifestyle requires them to make unpalatable changes in the 'here and now' for an uncertain benefit in the future.

→

- Perceptions of barriers to healthy lifestyles are more important than actual barriers; what is insurmountable for one individual will not be a problem for another.
- Self-efficacy is key to successful behavioural change; if you believe you can change you are far more likely to succeed.
- Self-regulation involves the setting of goals, but failing to achieve goals can put people at greater risk of excessive consumption. Goal setting requires a delicate balance to arrive at a sufficiently challenging but realistic goal.
- Implementation intentions can help people achieve their goals by providing strategies to deal with settings where the undesired behaviour is an ingrained habitual response to the situation.
- Social support is complex but indisputably related to health. It is possible, but not yet established, that health professionals and/or support groups could provide useful social support for behavioural change.
- The stage of change that an individual is in may influence their response to an intervention.
- The aim of motivational interviewing is to increase an individual's motivation to change.

Further resources

Thirlaway, K.J. and Upton, D. (2009). *The Psychology of Lifestyle: Promoting Healthy Behaviour*. London: Routledge.

Conner, M. and Norman, P. (2005). *Predicting Health Behaviour*. Berkshire: Open University Press.

Useful Web link

Change4life 0300 123 4567 http://www.nhs.uk/Change4Life

References

Aarts, H., Paulussen, T. and Schaalma, H. (1997). Physical exercise habit: On the conceptualization and formation of habitual health behaviours. *Health Education Research*, 21, 363–374.

Bandura, A. (1997). *Self-Efficacy. The Exercise of Control*. New York: WH Freeman.

Bandura, A. (1998). Health promotion from the perspective of social cognitive theory. *Psychology and Health*, 13, 623–649.

Barrientos-Gutierrez, T., Gimeno, D., Mangiane, T.W., Harrist, R.B. and Amick, B.C. (2007). Drinking social norms and drinking behaviours. *Occupational and Environmental Medicine*, 64, 602–608.

Blaxter, M. (1990). *Health and Lifestyles*. London: Sage.

Cabinet Office Strategy Unit. (2002). *Risk: Improving Government Capability to Handle Risk and Uncertainty*. London: Cabinet Office.

Conner, M. and Norman, P. (2005). *Predicting Health Behaviour,* 2nd ed. Berkshire: Open University Press.

Connolly, T., Arkes, H.R. and Hammond, K.R. (2000). *Judgement and Decision Making: An Interdisciplinary Reader*. Cambridge: Cambridge University Press.

Department of Health. (1999). *Saving Lives: Our Healthier Nation*. London: The Stationery Office.

Dilorio, C., Dudley, W.N., Kelly, M., Soet, J., Mbwara, J. and Sharpe Potter, J. (2001). Social cognitive correlates of sexual experience and condom use amoung 13 though 15 year old adolescents. *Journal of Adolescent Health, 29,* 208-216.

Faryna, E. and Morales, E. (2000). Self-efficacy and HIV-related risk behaviours among multi-ethnic adolescents. *Cultural Diversity and Ethnic Minority Psychology, 6*(1), 42-56.

Godin, G. and Kok, G. (1996). The theory of planned behaviour: A review of its applications to health-related behaviours. *American Journal of Health Promotion, 11,* 87-98.

Gollwitzer, P.M. and Sheeran, P. (2006). Implementation intentions and goal achievement: A meta-analysis of effects and processes. *Advances in Experimental Social Psychology, 38,* 69-119.

Gruber, K.J. (2008). Social support for exercise and dietary habits among college students. *Adolescence, 43*(171), 557-575.

Hagger, M.S., Chatzisarantis, N.L.D. and Biddle, S.J.H. (2002). A meta-analytic review of the theories of reasoned action and planned behaviour in physical activity: Predictive validity and the contribution of additional variables. *Journal of Sport and Exercise Psychology, 24,* 3-32.

Herman, C.P. and Polivy, J. (2004). The self-regulation of eating: Theoretical and practical problems. In *Handbook of Self Regulation: Research, Theory and Applications*. R.F. Baumeister and K.D. Vohs (eds). London. The Guilford Press.

Ismail, K., Thomas, S.M., Maissi, E., Chalder, T., Schmidt, U., Barlett, J., Patel, A., Dickens, C.M., Creed, F. and Treasure, J. (2008). Motivational enhancement therapy with and without cognitive behaviour therapy to treat type 1 diabetes. *Annals of Internal Medicine, 149,* 708-719.

Janis, I.L. (1968). *The Contours of Fear*. London: John Wiley & Sons.

Jeffery, R.W. and French, S.A. (1996). Socioeconomic status and weight control practices among 20 to 45 year old women. *American Journal of Public Health, 86*(7), 1005-1010.

Jones, A., Bentham, G., Foster, C., Hillsdon, M. and Panter, J. (2007). *Tackling Obesities: Future Choices - Obesogenic Environments - Evidence Review*. London: United Kingdom Government Foreign Programmes Office of Science and Innovation. Crown Copyright.

Kuther, T.L. and Timoshin, A. (2003). A comparision of social cognitive and psychosocial predictors of alcohol use by college students. *Journal of College Student Development, 44,* 143-154.

Lawton, J. (2002). Colonising the future: Temporal perceptions and health-relevant behaviors across the adult lifecourse. *Sociology of Health and Illness, 24,* 714-733.

Lawton, R. and Conner, M. (2007). Beyond cognition: Predicting health risk behaviours from instrumental and affective beliefs. *Health Pschology, 26,* 259-267.

Miller, W.R. and Rollnick, S. (2002). Motivational interviewing: Preparing people for change, 2nd edn. New York: Guilford Press.

Mutrie, N., Carney, C., Blamey, A., Crawford, F., Aitchison, T. and Whitelaw, A. (2002). 'Walk in to work out': A randomised controlled trial of a self help intervention to promote active commuting. *Journal of Epidemiology and Community Health,* 56, 407-412.

Nabi, R.L. (2002). Discrete emotions and persuasion. In J.P. Dillard and M. Pfau (eds) *The Persuasion Handbook: Developments in Theory and Practice.* London: Sage.

Nigg, C.R., Borrelli, B., Maddock, J. and Dishman, R.K. (2008). A theory of physical activity maintenance. *Applied Psychology: An international review,* 57(4), 544-560.

Orford, J. (2001). *Excessive Appetites: A Psychological View of Addictions,* 2nd edn. Chichester: John Wiley and Sons.

Pirie, P., Rooney, B., Pechacek, T., Lando, H. and Schmid, L. (1997). Incorporating social support into a community-wide smoking cessation contest. *Addictive Behaviour,* 22(1), 131-137.

Plant, M. and Plant, M. (2006). *Binge Britain.* Oxford: Oxford University Press.

Rasmussen, H.N., Wrosch, C., Scheier, M.F. and Carver, C.S. (2006). Self-regulation processes and health: The importance of optimism and goal adjustment. *Journal of Personality,* 74(6), 1721-1747.

Rigby, K., Brown, M., Anagnostou, P., Ross, M.W. and Rosser, B.P.S. (1989). Shock tactics to counter AIDS: The Australian Experience. *Psychology and Health,* 3, 145-159.

Rovniak, L.S., Anderson, E.S., Winett, R.A. and Stephens, R.S. (2002). Social cognitive determinants of physical activity in young adults: A prospective structural equation analysis. *Annals of Behavioural Medicine,* 24, 149-156.

Strecher, V.J., Seijts, G.H., Kok, G.J., Latham, G.P., Glasgow, R., DeVellis, B., Meertens, R.M. and Bulger, D.W. (1995). Goal setting as a strategy for health behaviour change. *Health Education Quarterly,* 22(2), 190-200.

Sutton, S. (1982). Fear-arousing communications: A critical examination of theory and research. In J.R. Eiser (ed) *Social Psychology and Behavioural Medicine.* London: Wiley, pp. 303-337.

Swinburn, B., Figger, G. and Raza, F. (1999). Dissecting obesogenic environments: The development and application of a framework for identifying and prioritising environmental interventions for obesity. *American Journal of Preventive Medicine,* 29, 563-570.

Thirlaway, K.J. and Heggs, D. (2005). Interpreting risk messages: Women's responses to a health story. *Health, Risk and Society,* 7, 107-121.

Thirlaway, K.J. and Upton, D. (2009). *The Psychology of Lifestyle: Promoting Healthy Behaviour.* London: Routledge.

Wang, H.X., Mittleman, M.A. and Orth-Gomer, K. (2005). Influence of social support on progression of coronary heart disease in women. *Social Science and Medicine,* 60, 599-607.

Walker, J. (2001). *Control and the Psychology of Health.* Buckingham: Open University Press.

Weinstein, N.D. (1984). Why it won't happen to me: Perceptions of risk factors and susceptibility. *Health Psychology,* 3, 431-457.

Westbrook, D., Kennedy, H. and Krik, J. (2007). *An Introduction to Cognitive Behavioural Therapy.* London: Sage.

Chapter 3
Eating well

LEARNING OBJECTIVES

At the end of this chapter you will:

- Be able to identify definitions of a healthy diet
- Describe the extent of the obesity problem in the UK at present
- Have explored the consequences of poor diet and obesity for the individual
- Identify various methods of assessing diet and eating behaviour and be aware of the limitations of each approach
- Understand the impact of psychosocial and environmental factors on diet and eating behaviour
- Be able to analyse the extent to which interventions aimed at increasing healthy eating are successful

Case study

Robert is a 28-year-old man who works in the finance office of a large supermarket chain. Bob, as he likes to be called, has been working in an office since completing his accountancy degree a few years ago. Bob always had a problem with his weight, but since his son was born some five years ago his weight has ballooned and he now tips the scales at 23 stone (or 146 kilos). He has found that access to a regular wage packet, limited exercise, regular nights out and access to a plentiful supply of food (he has a staff discount) mean that he has put on considerable weight.

Bob is married and currently has a five-year-old son, Dave, although he and his wife are trying for another child. His wife is also obese and they fear that their weight is getting in the way of them having another child. Dave is rather chubby and takes a great delight in eating fish fingers and chips to the exclusion of most other food!

→

Bob now finds that his regular diet of takeaways and pre-packaged meals with lim-ited fruit and vegetables is leading him on a downward spiral. He used to play five-a-side football with 'the lads', but given his weight and because he becomes out of breath easily he has stopped playing, merely turning up for the post-match drinking session.

Bob has recently had a health scare; he had a pain in the centre of his chest and was rushed to hospital where he was admitted overnight for observation. This caused great family concern and started to get them all to worry about their lifestyle. Although the hospital tests revealed no significant problems, his blood pressure was high (160/100 mmHg) and his BMI (44) placed him in the morbidly obese category. He was referred to you to try to reduce his weight and improve his overall weight control.

Discussion point

How would you address Bob's eating behaviour and work with him and his family to try to reduce his weight and ensure that he maintains a healthy diet?

Introduction

Unlike many of the other behaviours (e.g. smoking or drinking alcohol) highlighted in this text, we all eat and we all have to eat. Eating can have a protective benefit; for example, eating a healthy diet protects from a third of all cancers, diabetes, osteoporosis, heart dis-ease, strokes and tooth decay. In contrast, having an unhealthy diet can lead to considerable health damage, such as osteoporosis, heart disease and cancer. It is estimated that obesity is responsible for more than 9,000 premature deaths per year in England, and a similar propor-tion in Scotland, Wales and Northern Ireland (Canoy and Buchan, 2007). Forecast estimates suggest that moving towards the recommended diet could result in significant benefits in terms of both mortality and morbidity (see Table 3.1).

Table 3.1 Premature mortality and morbidity improvements resulting from move towards recommended diets

	Premature mortality avoided	Quality adjusted life years (QALYs) gained
Increase fruit and vegetable intake by 136 g/day	42,000	411,000
Reduce daily salt intake from average 9 g to 6 g	20,000	170,000
Cut saturated fat intake by 2.5% of energy	3,500	33,000
Cut added sugar intake by 1.75% of energy	3,500	49,000

Source: Ofcom (2006)

Government recommendations

The national guidelines suggest that a healthy diet is a balanced diet based on five major food groups: breads, other cereals and potatoes; fruit and vegetables; milk and dairy foods; meat, fish and alternatives; and foods containing fats and sugars (see Photograph 3.1). The Department of Health (1999) defines good nutrition in the 'Saving Lives: Our Healthier Nation' document as '. . . plenty of fruit and vegetables, cereals, and not too much fatty and salty food'. Although this definition is hardly specific, government and policy makers have continued with the concept of an 'eatwell plate' (see Photograph 3.1).

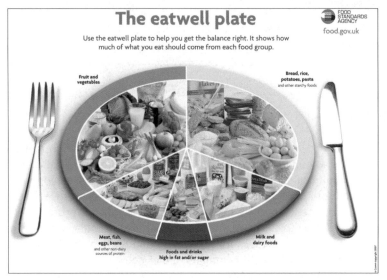

Photograph 3.1 Balance of a good diet
Source: From Food Standards Agency, http://www.eatwell.gov.uk/healthydiet/eatwellplate/?lang=en, © Crown copyright 2007. Crown copyright material is reproduced with permission under the terms of the Click-Use Licence

In addition to this general 'eat well' guidance, there are two specific government recommendations: eat at least five portions of fruit and vegetables per day, and reduce consumption of salt to a maximum of 6 g per day. One of the major recommendations, and the one that has been the focus of much marketing and advertising, is that at least five portions of fruit and vegetables are consumed each day (World Health Organization (WHO), 2004), with a portion being approximately 80 g (e.g. one medium apple, or three heaped tablespoons of peas).

Applying this to Bob

Does Bob eat five portions of fruit and vegetables per day? Would his salt intake be within recommended guidelines?

Evidence from the National Diet and Nutrition Survey found that the average consumption of fruit and vegetables was less than three portions per adult per day. Only 13% of men and 15% of women consumed the recommended five or more portions a day (Henderson *et al.*, 2002). Social class differences are also apparent, with those in the working class consuming 50% less than those in professional groups. A particular area of concern is children's diet – research suggests that nearly 20% of those aged between 4 and 18 years eat no fruit at all during a typical week (Strategy Unit, 2008). Despite considerable effort, increased marketing commitment and expenditure towards increasing the consumption of fruit and vegetables, there has been little success (Strategy Unit, 2008).

Given the extent of the obesity problem in the UK and the potential health difficulties associated with this, it is not surprising that the UK government (along with the separate legislatures) has developed strategic plans to counteract the looming difficulties. For example, The Food and Health Action Plan and the Activity Coordination Team is a cross-government group (led by the Department of Health) to improve public health through better diet. Examples of such action include:

Breastfeeding: action to encourage more women to breastfeed and to continue for at least six months.

Reform of the Welfare Food Scheme: to ensure children in poverty have access to a healthy diet and increased support for breastfeeding.

5 A DAY programme: including the National School Fruit Scheme.

Food in Schools Programme: promoting a 'whole school approach' and encouraging greater access to healthier choices within schools.

Work with the food industry: to address the amount of fat, salt and added sugar in the diet (with the Food Standards Agency).

New GP contract: practices will be required to offer relevant health promotion advice to patients.

Banning 'junk food' advertising: As of January 2007, the independent regulator for the communications industry, Ofcom, placed a total ban on adverts for foods high in fat, salt and sugar during all preschool children's programmes, all programmes on mainstream channels aimed at children, all cable and satellite children's channels, and programmes aimed at young people, such as music shows and general entertainment programmes which would appeal to a 'higher than average' number of under-16s.

Health consequences of a poor diet

A poor diet can contribute to a range of illnesses, including both coronary heart disease (CHD) and cancer (see Table 3.2). A poor diet can also result in increased falls and fractures

Table 3.2 Diseases associated with obesity

Cardiovascular disease

Cancer

Diabetes

Stroke

Hypertension

Angina

Dental decay

Table 3.3 Health risks associated with lack of dietary elements

	Found in	Health risk
Vitamin A	Liver, cheese, eggs and oily fish	Weakening of immune system
Vitamin B6	Poultry, whole cereals and peanuts	Depression and irritability
Vitamin B12	Meat, salmon, cheese and eggs	Anaemia
Vitamin C	Oranges, peppers, broccoli, cabbage	Bleeding gums, aching joints
Vitamin D	Oily fish, eggs	Muscle weakness and aching bones
Calcium	Milk, cheese, broccoli and cabbage	Bone and tooth decay
Folic acid	Broccoli, Brussel sprouts, peas, brown rice	Anaemia
Iron	Meat, bones, whole grains and watercress	Anaemia
Magnesium	Spinach, nuts, bread	Tiredness and bone and tooth decay
Vitamin B3	Beef, pork, eggs and milk	Skin problems, dizziness, swelling of tongue
Potassium	Bananas, vegetables, nuts	Irregular heartbeat, irritability and nausea
Vitamin B2	Mushrooms, rice, eggs and milk	Skin problems, difficulty sleeping
Vitamin B1	Peas and other vegetables, pork, milk and cheese	Headaches and tiredness
Zinc	Meat, shellfish, milk and cheese	Hair loss, skin problems, diarrhoea

in older people, low birth weight, increased childhood morbidity and mortality, and increased dental cavities in children (see Table 3.3 for links between specific nutrient deficits and poor health). There is also evidence to support the link between poor diet and anti-social behaviour, not to mention growing concern over the economic implications of the population's weight gain.

The benefits of an improved diet have been highlighted in a number of public health documents and government policies. For example:

- Reducing cholesterol levels by just 10% would prevent some 25,000 deaths every year (Unal *et al.*, 2004), which could be achieved by reducing saturated fat intake.

- The incidence of strokes could be decreased by increasing the consumption of fruit and vegetables.

- Hypertension could be reduced by reducing the salt intake and therefore have a positive impact on the incidence of cardiovascular diseases such as CHD/stroke (Davis *et al.*, 2000).

- Approximately 40% of endometrial cancer and 10% of breast and colon cancers would be avoided by maintaining a healthy weight (i.e. BMI of 25 or less).

- Increased dietary fibre is associated with a decreased risk of colorectal and pancreatic cancer.

Key message

Healthy eating brings with it considerable health benefits.

Obesity may be a risk factor in a number of chronic diseases such as heart disease, stroke, some cancers and type 2 diabetes (Zaninotto *et al.*, 2006). National Audit Office (NAO, 2001) figures suggest that if there were one million fewer obese people in this country, this would lead to around 15,000 fewer people with CHD, 34,000 fewer people developing type 2 diabetes and 99,000 fewer people with high blood pressure. Greater awareness of the disease burden associated with obesity has led to concern over the economic implications of the population's weight gain. The Health Select Committee (2006, as cited in McPherson *et al.*, 2007) has estimated that the cost of obesity is £3.3–3.7 billion per year and of obesity plus overweight £6.6–7.4 billion. Based on Foresight extrapolations to 2050, the potential combined direct and indirect costs of obesity in the UK could rise to £52 billion per year (at today's prices) (McPherson *et al.*, 2007).

The consequences of a poor diet are more than just obesity. For example, it has been suggested that around 30% of all cancer deaths can be attributed to smoking cigarettes – but around 35% can be attributable, in some part, to a poor diet (Doll and Peto, 1981). A diet involving significant intake of high-fat foods, high levels of salt and low levels of fibre appears to be particularly implicated (World Cancer Research Fund, 1997). In addition to cancer, excessive fat intake has been implicated in disease and death from several serious illnesses, including CHD. According to the Food Standards Agency (FSA, 2004), 73,000 cardiovascular deaths and 34,000 other deaths a year are related to the type and quantity of the food we eat. Obesity is an important issue in the poverty–poor diet–poor health cycle. A study (Rayner and Scarborough, 2005) estimated that food-related ill-health is responsible for about 10% of morbidity and mortality in the UK. The researchers concluded that the cost to the health service of dealing with poor dietary habits was significantly higher than the estimate for the annual cost of smoking, which is around £1.5 billion. They estimated that food accounts for costs of £6 billion a year (9% of the NHS budget). It should be emphasised that this chapter will explore the obesity 'epidemic' and this side of the diet equation rather than the malnutrition side of a poor diet (although the latter has been suggested as costing the

NHS some £7.3 billion a year, i.e. higher than the cost of obesity; Rayner and Scarborough, 2005).

Applying this to Bob

What health problems may Bob be facing because of his current diet and eating patterns?

Obviously, eating the right foods can prevent illness and promote health. For example, eating fruit and vegetables may offer protection against some forms of cancer (e.g. bowel). Block *et al.* (1992) suggested that on the basis of 132 of 170 studies there is evidence to suggest that fruit and vegetables offer significant protection against cancer. Other studies have indicated that it is also of benefit for stroke and heart disease (Ness and Powles, 1997).

Assessment of diet

There are many ways of assessing diet, but the most easily employed within a clinical setting would be the recording of a food diary (see Table 3.4). In this case, the individual patient or client would be asked to record their daily intake of a range of foodstuffs (based on the five categories in the eatwell plate).

Applying this to Bob

On the basis of the case study presented at the start of the chapter, complete the food diary for Bob.

The other method of assessing the consequence of diet is to infer it from body measurements. The most common form of body measurement is the Body Mass Index (BMI). BMI is calculated using the equation weight (kg)/height (m^2) or can be read from a graph (see Figure 3.1). Although BMI is a good way of assessing body fat levels for the average person, there are problems when using this method to assess muscular people (overestimates possible) and the elderly (possible underestimate of true BMI). For example, athletes and well-trained body builders have a very low percentage of body fat, but their BMI may be in the overweight range. This is because BMI does not distinguish between fat mass and lean mass.

Key message

BMI is calculated by dividing weight (kg) by height squared (m^2).

Table 3.4 Your food diary

Think back over the last week. On how many days did you eat fruit, vegetables, fried food and high-fat dairy food? Fill in the table below.

Food type	How many days in a week do you eat this type of food?
Fruit (e.g. bananas, apples, mangoes, pears and plums) 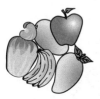	
Vegetables (carrots, peas, broccoli) 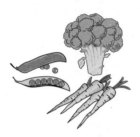	
Fried food (e.g. burgers, fried chips, chicken) 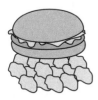	
High-fat dairy food (e.g. ice cream, full fat milk, cheese, butter) 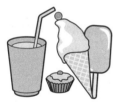	

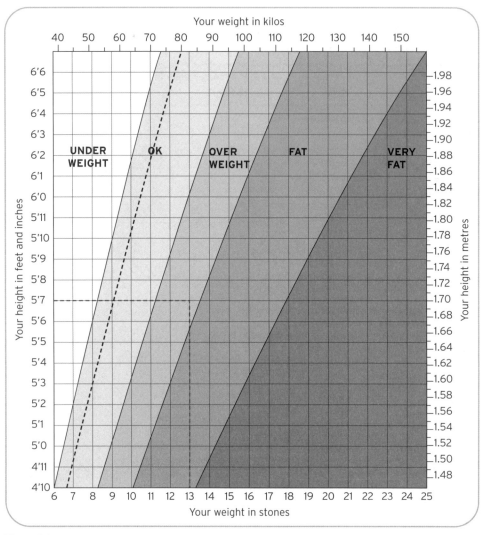

Figure 3.1 BMI measurements

For adults, BMI provides a simple guide to whether weight matches height appropriately. For children, however, BMI is more complex because weight varies with height as children grow. It is calculated the same way as for adults but then compared to typical values for other children of the same age and biological sex.

Discussion point

Calculate Bob's BMI. What level of risk is Bob at because of his BMI?

Using the UK National BMI percentile classification system for children aged 2-15 years, overweight and obesity are categorised as follows:

Description	BMI centile for child's exact age
Not overweight	85th centile or below
Overweight	Over 85th to 95th centile
Obese	95th centile or over

Although it is rather crude and imprecise, BMI is a useful measure of adiposity and correlates well with the risk of obesity-related diseases (Haslam and James, 2005). In many studies, BMI is calculated using self-report height and weight. However, a recent systematic review has demonstrated that this self-report BMI may be lower than a measured BMI, i.e. some obese individuals are being misclassified as being non-obese based on self-reported BMI (Connor Gorber *et al.*, 2007). Importantly, this self-report misclassification is not random: moderately obese individuals are more likely to side with non-obese than severely obese, the latter having a BMI which is further away from the obese/non-obese cut-off value. Consequently, you should always take recordings of height and weight rather than rely on self-report, as this may be an underestimate.

Key message

If possible, always measure height and weight – do not rely on self-report.

An alternative method for assessing body size is to measure waist circumference. Although most people can measure their own waist size, they usually do it at the smallest point rather than the appropriate place (see Table 3.5). The final method for assessing body shape is the waist-to-hip ratio (see Table 3.5). The waist-to-hip ratio is a simple measure of where fat is stored on the body. Most people store their body fat in two places: around their waist and around their hips. Storing extra weight around your waist (apple shaped) puts a person at a higher health risk than someone carrying extra weight around their hips and thighs (pear shaped). Waist-to-hip ratio is calculated by dividing the waist measurement by hip measurement.

Table 3.5 How to get waist and hip measurements

Use a measuring tape to take the waist and hip measurement:

Waist: This measurement should be taken at the smaller section of the natural waist, usually located just above the belly button.

Hips: Hip measurement should be taken at the hips on the widest part of your buttocks.

Healthy waist-to-hip ratios

A healthy waist-to-hip ratio for women is **0.8** or lower.

A healthy ratio for men is **1.0** or lower.

Ratios above **0.8** for women and **1.0** for men are associated with obesity and are linked to greater risk of health complications and diseases.

Table 3.6 Risk of associated disease according to BMI and waist size

BMI		Waist less than or equal to 40 in. (men) or 35 in. (women)	Waist greater than 40 in. (men) or 35 in. (women)
18.5 or less	Underweight	-	N/A
18.5-24.9	Normal	-	N/A
25.0-29.9	Overweight	Increased	High
30.0-34.9	Obese	High	Very high
35.0-39.9	Obese	Very high	Very high
40 or greater	Extremely obese	Extremely high	Extremely high

Both BMI and waist sizes come with cut-offs that suggest whether the individual has a problem with their size or not (see Table 3.6).

Why do people eat unhealthily?

There have been a number of explanations for why people eat what they do, and these have ranged from the genetic through to the social-environmental, taking in media and cognitive factors along the way. Although it is impossible in this brief review to cover all these different proposals, it is worth exploring some of them to examine how they translate into interventions.

The media

The media is often cited as one of the major reasons for the increase in diet problems in the developed world (Boyce, 2007). There have been a number of studies that have linked TV viewing and childhood obesity, with the common conclusion being that television viewing is an 'important contributing factor to childhood obesity' (Hancox and Poulton, 2006, p. 171). There are a number of potential explanations for this link, but two predominate. On the one hand, it may be that watching TV encourages a sedentary lifestyle. Alternatively, it may be that media advertising promotes unhealthy consumption, and research has confirmed that this may be the case (Ofcom, 2004).

Obesogenic environments

The term 'obesogenic environment' was coined by Swinburn et al. (1999) who argued that the physical, economic, social and cultural environments of the developed world promote positive energy balance (i.e. calorie intake exceeding calorie output) and consequently weight gain and obesity. Examples of environmental influences that may encourage us to eat more than we need include the marketing of energy-dense drinks and snacks, for example through television advertising and vending machines in schools, and the increase in portion sizes where an average meal may provide up to 2,000 kcal - almost the entire recommended daily intake for most adults. Time constraints on workers have led to an increase in demand for convenience food, pre-packaged foods with short preparation times, and in food consumption away from the home. This has also led to a decrease in structured meals and an increase in snacking which is often (although not always) densely calorific, along with the emergence of fast-food restaurants which are associated with a high-fat diet.

Applying this to Bob

How does Bob's environment contribute to his weight gain and poor diet?

Psychosocial factors

Some key social factors associated with a poor diet include:

Low income and debt: Healthier foods are generally more expensive than the less healthy alternatives. Fresh fruit and vegetables are less affordable.

Poor accessibility to affordable healthy foods: Many local shops are closing and being replaced with larger, out-of-town stores. This is particularly an issue in deprived areas where such developments mean that there are increased costs within the local shops, poor-quality foodstuffs and less choice remaining in the locality. The out-of-town public stores may have poor transport links and consequently not be as easily accessible as the local shops with poor-quality and expensive food.

Factors involved in food production and the food chain: The cheap nutrient level of easily available foodstuffs such as TV-dinners may contain high fat, sugar or salt content.

Poor literacy and numeracy skills: These are barriers to maintaining a healthy diet, household budget, management and employment.

Food labelling: The recently introduced food labelling agreement means that more information is available to the consumer. However, there is still some disagreement about the nature of the information provided and the value derived by the consumer from the information.

Food marketing: Adverts to children usually focus on food that is high in fat or sugar. Consequently, the government is introducing new restrictions on what can be advertised and marketed to young children. However, there is still doubt about the finer details of this approach and, given its recent introduction, its success is yet to be assessed.

Key message

There are a range of psychosocial factors that can impact on eating behaviour.

Box 3.1 Applying research in practice

Reducing children's television viewing to prevent obesity: a randomised controlled trial (Robinson, 1999)

The aim of this experiment was to assess the effects of reducing television, videotape and video game use on changes in adiposity, physical activity and dietary intake. Participants were 192 primary school pupils from two socio-demographically and scholastically matched schools (mean age 8.9 years).

One school was randomly assigned to receive the intervention while the other was assigned an assessments-only control. Children in the intervention group received an 18-lesson, 6-month classroom curriculum based on Bandura's social cognitive theory (1986). Early lessons included self-monitoring and self-reporting of television viewing, videotape and video game use to motivate children to reduce the time they spent on these activities.

Compared to controls, children in the intervention group had significant decreases in body mass index, tricep skin fold thickness, waist circumference and waist-to-hip ratio. Relative to controls, intervention group changes were accompanied by significant decreases in children's reported television viewing, meals eaten in front of the television and video game use.

Key message

Reducing television, videotape and video game use may be a promising population-based approach to prevent childhood obesity.

Models of eating behaviour

One core theoretical psychological perspective of why people have unhealthy diets is the developmental approach, which suggests that food preferences are learned in childhood and can be understood in terms of exposure, social learning and associative learning.

Developmental approach

For infants and children, eating is typically a social event and others can have a considerable impact on children's food preferences and food selections. Hence, from a social learning perspective, it would be suggested that children's preferences for and consumption of disliked vegetables were enhanced when children observed peers selecting and eating foods that the observing child disliked. Parental behaviour and attitudes are central to the process of social learning; however, this association is not straightforward, as parents often differentiate between themselves and their children in terms of food-related motivations and food choice. Promise of a reward is a time-honoured parental tactic for promoting consumption of healthy food. Nevertheless, it has been argued that treating food consumption in this way may actually decrease liking for that food. Birch (1999, p. 53) concluded that:

> . . . although these practices can induce children to eat more vegetables in the short run, evidence from our research suggests that in the long run parental control attempts

may have negative effects on the quality of children's diets by reducing their prefer-ences for those foods.

The developmental model emphasises the importance of learning and focuses on the development of food preferences in childhood. From this perspective, eating behaviour is influenced by exposure, social learning and associative learning.

Applying this to Bob

How could Bob's behaviour impact on Dave's diet?

Key message

Promoting healthy eating at an early age can have a long-term positive impact.

Cognitive approach

Cognitive models of eating behaviour explore the extent to which cognitions predict and explain behaviour. Most research from a cognitive perspective has drawn on social cognition models, and several models have been developed (see Chapter 7 for details on some of these models); the Health Belief Model (HBM: Becker and Rosenstock, 1984), Protection Motivation Theory (PMT: Rogers, 1985), Health Action Process Approach (HAPA: Schwarzer, 1992), Theory of Reasoned Action (TRA: Fishbein and Ajzen, 1975) and its descendant the Theory of Planned Behaviour (TPB: Ajzen, 1985). All five models share the assumption that attitudes and beliefs are major determinants of eating behaviour; however, they vary in terms of the cognitions they include and whether they use behavioural intentions or actual behaviour as their outcome measure.

These cognitive models of eating behaviour explore the extent to which cognitions predict and explain behaviour. Cognitive models are not only informative with regard to their ability to predict behaviour, but also provide a helpful insight into ways of influencing this behaviour (Stroebe and Stroebe, 1995).

Key message

Attitudes and beliefs influence our eating behaviour.

Improving diet

The National Institute for Health and Clinical Excellence (NICE) (2007) have recently pub-lished a set of generic principles that can be used as the basis for planning and delivering interventions aimed at changing health-related behaviours. The guidance is for healthcare professionals with direct or indirect responsibility for helping people to change their health behaviour. NICE recommend that practitioners working with individuals should select interventions that motivate and support people to:

- understand the short- medium- and longer-term consequences of their health-related behaviours, for themselves and others;
- feel positive about the benefits of health-enhancing behaviours and changing their behaviour;
- plan their changes in terms of easy steps over time;
- recognise how their social contexts and relationships may affect their behaviour, and identify and plan for situations that might undermine the changes they are trying to make;
- plan explicit 'if-then' coping strategies to prevent relapse;
- make a personal commitment to adopt health-enhancing behaviours by setting (and recording) goals to undertake clearly defined behaviours, in particular contexts, over a specified time;
- share their behaviour change goals with others.

This guidance should be read in conjunction with other health guidance issued by NICE. For example, NICE (2006) have published specific recommendations on how to increase the effectiveness of interventions to improve diet and reduce energy intake. In this case, NICE recommend that dietary interventions should:

- be multi-component (i.e. including dietary modification, targeted advice, family involvement and goal setting);
- be tailored to the individual;
- provide ongoing support;
- include behaviour change strategies;
- include awareness-raising promotional activities as part of a longer-term, multi-component intervention rather than a one-off activity.

Hence, the healthcare professional needs to be aware of the interventions that are available – whether they be structural, psychological or medical. A number of interventions have been developed and implemented to improve diet and eating behaviours. These have been at both individual and population level. Those that are most relevant to the practising healthcare professional are presented here. How they can be implemented with individuals will be described so that essential tips can be appreciated.

Food Dudes

The first intervention described, Food Dudes, aims to prevent dietary problems. The aim is to introduce an educational programme for primary school children to encourage them to eat healthily from an early age. Despite considerable efforts over a number of years, there is limited evidence to suggest that educational approaches to dietary change (that is, providing basic information about what constitutes a 'healthy' diet) alter children's eating habits (Department of Health, 2005; Bajekal et al., 2003). Clearly, even if children do know what they should be eating, this does not necessarily translate into their dietary behaviour. In light

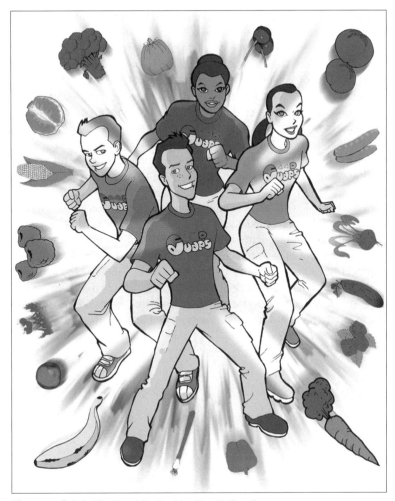

Photograph 3.2 The Food Dudes Healthy Eating Programme
Source: University of Wales, Bangor

of such evidence, a group of psychologists from the University of Bangor developed the Food Dudes Programme (see Photograph 3.2) based on underlying psychological principles.

Based on the principles of the Food Dudes programme, the key elements of any intervention would include the following:

- The earlier a child is exposed to different foodstuffs, the better the outcome.
- Model positive eating behaviour at home, at school and in leisure.
- Increase the range of food to which children are exposed.
- Reward increasing choice and healthy eating.
- Educate about healthy eating.
- Ensure that the home and school environment encourages healthy eating.

The Food Dudes Programme is specifically designed for 4–11-year-olds to encourage the consumption of fruit and vegetables. The theoretical position of the programme is primarily based on research into learning and cognitive processes, in particular peer modelling and rewards (Horne *et al.*, 2004). Children watch a series of fun video episodes featuring the Food Dudes, a group of positive-role-model kids who gain superpowers when they eat fruit and vegetables. The children are then given the opportunity to taste fruit and vegetables themselves. If they succeed in consuming these foods, a variety of Food Dudes stickers and prizes are given out as rewards. There is also a home pack to support the programme which includes a diary to record fruit and vegetable consumption, plus tips and advice on healthy eating. By encouraging children to taste fruit and vegetables repeatedly, the programme helps them to discover the intrinsically rewarding properties of the foods. In the process, they also come to think of themselves as fruit and vegetable eaters in a school culture that is now strongly supportive of healthy eating (The Food Dudes Healthy Eating Programme, 2006).

Initial evaluation of the Food Dudes programme showed that it resulted in large, statistically significant increases in fruit and vegetable consumption at snack time and lunch time for both boys and girls in infant and junior schools (Lowe *et al.*, 2001, 2002). Successive studies have demonstrated that these positive effects are not confined to the foods experienced during the programme, but spread to a wide range of other fruit and vegetables. Similarly, the positive effects have been found to be general across contexts. For example, increased fruit and vegetable consumption at school was reflected by increased consumption at home. What's more, in one follow-up study, increases in fruit and vegetable consumption still persisted 15 months after the end of the intervention, highlighting the programme's long-term effectiveness (Lowe *et al.*, 2007).

Key message

Introducing new foods to children can widen their choice of foods and encourage healthy eating.

Applying this to Bob

If Bob started to have a wider selection of foods from which Dave could choose, and these were positively reinforced by Bob and his wife, this might lead to improved eating habits.

Box 3.2 Applying research in practice

Promoting children's fruit and vegetable consumption: Interventions using the Theory of Planned Behaviour as a framework (Gratton *et al.*, 2007)

The objectives of this longitudinal study were threefold; i) to assess the effectiveness of a motivation-based intervention derived from the Theory of Planned Behaviour on children's fruit and vegetable consumption, ii) to assess the effectiveness of a volition-based intervention using the formation of implementation intentions on children's fruit and vegetable consumption, and iii) to compare the effectiveness of each intervention.

→

One hundred and ninety-eight children from a secondary school in the UK were randomly allocated to a control group or one of two intervention groups. Theory of Planned Behaviour variables and fruit and vegetable consumption were assessed at the beginning of the study and again two weeks later. Intervention group A formed an implementation intention stating how, when and where they could eat five portions of fruit and vegetables a day, while intervention group B stated ways in which they could overcome motivational barriers to eating five portions a day.

Both interventions significantly increased fruit and vegetable consumption compared to baseline. However, the volitional intervention was the only one to increase consumption significantly over the control, suggesting that it was more effective at changing behaviour.

Key message

It is possible to change children's eating behaviour.

Prescriptions for fruit and vegetables

At the level of the health practitioner, Kearney *et al.*, (2005) report on a brief preventative intervention deployed in primary care consultations in a deprived area in North West England. At the centre of the scheme is a prescription for fruit and vegetables which GPs, nurses, health visitors and midwives issue to patients on an opportunistic basis. Each prescription contains four vouchers offering a £1 discount when £3 or more is spent on fruit and vegetables. As the health professionals issue the prescription they link it explicitly to key five-a-day messages. Early feedback suggested that that the intervention was successful in highlighting to patients the connection between food and health. Furthermore, clinicians expressed satisfaction with having a simple preventative intervention which could be deployed quickly (1-2 minutes) and effectively during routine primary care consultations.

Primary care remains the public's preferred source of food and health information. It provides a natural setting for health promotion, which is usually long term and characterised by trust. Hence, all primary care consultations should be accompanied by some health promotion message, whether this be about diet, weight, smoking or alcohol.

Discussion point

What sort of health promotion should primary care be involved in? How can you change your practice to promote healthy eating?

Although such food prescriptions can be useful and encourage a more focused approach to dietary selection, there are psychological principles that will help explain why a person succeeds in changing their diet, and why they ask for assistance in the first place. One important concept that has been highlighted throughout this text is the concept of self-efficacy.

Self-efficacy

One of the most important concepts when looking at the success of psychological interventions is the concept of self-efficacy (French *et al.*,1996; Dennis and Goldberg, 1996). Self-efficacy regarding weight loss (Rodin *et al.*, 1988), the ability to handle emotions, life situations (Jeffrey *et al.*, 1984) and exercise have been related to later weight loss maintenance. Follow-up data on weight maintainers have also shown that they have more confidence in their ability to manage their weight than weight regainers (DePue *et al.*, 1995). More information on self-efficacy is presented in Chapter 4.

> **Key message**
>
> An individual's belief in their chances of success in changing their behaviour is key.

Decisional balance

One way to prompt individuals into making a change is to encourage them to consider the **pros** and the **cons** of changing their behaviour. Pros and cons were originally derived from Janis and Mann's (1977) model of decision making and have become critical constructs in the transtheoretical, or stages of change, model. The balance between the pros and cons varies depending on which stage of change the individual is in. However, change is unlikely to occur until the reasons for change outweigh the reasons for staying the same.

When thinking about change, most of us don't really consider all 'sides' in a logical way. Instead, we often do what we think we 'should' do, avoid doing things we don't feel like doing, or just feel confused or overwhelmed and give up thinking about it at all. Thinking through the pros and cons of changing or not changing is one way to help us make sure we have fully considered the consequences of our behaviour. This can help us to 'hang on' to our plan in times of stress or temptation.

Using the material in Table 3.7, a list of the pros and cons associated with changing diet or eating behaviour can be made. For most people, 'making a change' will probably mean eating

Table 3.7 Decisional balance sheet

	Benefits/Pros	Costs/Cons
Making a change		
Not changing		

healthily, but it is important to state the *specific* changes that individuals might want to make, e.g. cutting down on saturated fat and sugar, eating five portions of fruit and vegetables a day or trying to eat less salt – no more than 6 g a day.

Applying this to Bob

What sort of costs and benefits would you imagine Bob would list in his decisional balance sheet?

Goal setting

Once the individual has made the decision that they want to change their behaviour and they want to start eating healthily, it is important for them to be given specific goals. It is of limited value if you suggest that the individual 'loses weight' or 'eats more healthily'; the guidance must be specific – 'lose two kilos', or 'start to eat five portions of fruit and vegetables per day'. In this way, the goals need to be SMART (that is, **S**pecific, **M**easurable, **A**chievable, **R**ealistic and **T**imed):

Specific: Specific goals are essential to diet improvement programmes. They represent the difference in focus and motivation between 'I should lose some weight' and 'I'm going to lose a kilo a week for the next seven weeks – this means in seven weeks' time I'll be 7 kilos lighter'.

Measurable: The starting point, the weight goal and milestones along the way are all required so that progress can be checked at regular intervals in order to maintain confidence and ensure the plan is on track.

Achievable: It must be possible to achieve the goal; this is the key to success. If the goals are large – losing two or more stone – then the goals should be broken down into smaller steps, an initial goal of half a stone for example. A new milestone goal can then be set once you have achieved your first goal.

Realistic: There's no point attempting to be half a stone lighter by the end of next week. Even if it were possible it would be setting the client up for failure in the longer term.

Timed: Setting a time frame for the goal gives the client a clear target to work towards. Remember, the time frame must be measurable, achievable and realistic!

Applying this to Bob

Prepare some SMART targets for both Bob and Dave.

You need to develop these goals in conjunction with the client and the client should be asked:

What are you going to do?

How are you going to do it?

Where are you going to do it?

When are you going to do it?

With whom are you going to do it?

Once the goals are set, the process outlined in Figure 3.2 can be followed.

Key message

SMART targets are essential in promoting behaviour change.

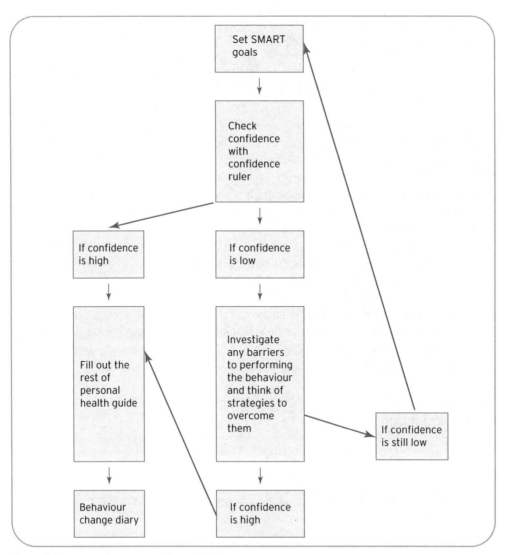

Figure 3.2 Process for encouraging weight loss

Changing diet through motivational interviewing

The technique described in Figure 3.2 is based on the stages of change model and using a motivational interviewing technique. Motivational interviewing is a directive, client-centred counselling technique for enhancing intrinsic motivation. Motivational interviewing works by helping the patient to articulate why it is important for them to change and by increasing their self-efficacy so that they have the confidence to do so. It is usually used alongside the transtheoretical model (TTM) (Prochaska and DiClemente, 1983) which is discussed in much detail throughout this text. In short, the model suggests that change proceeds through a series of stages. The model (see Figure 3.3) is important as it allows the practitioner to iden-tify where individuals are in their behaviour; with this in mind, appropriate interventions can be developed and implemented. The five stages of change are:

1. *Pre-contemplation:* The patient has no intention of making any changes;
2. *Contemplation:* The patient is considering making some changes;

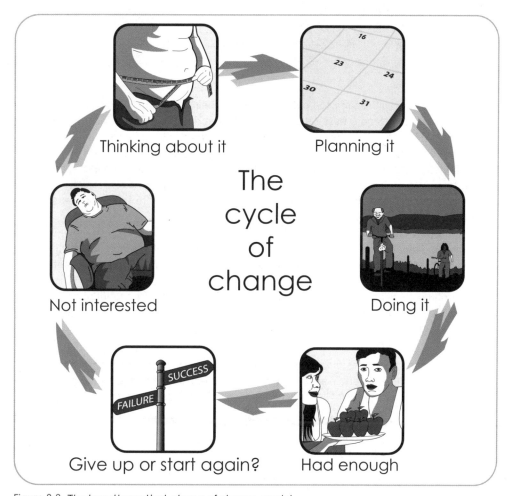

Figure 3.3 The transtheoretical, stages of change, model
Source: Prochaska *et al.* (1992)

3. *Preparation:* The patient is making small changes; has developed a plan of action and intends to initiate it in the near future

4. *Action:* The patient is actively participating in the new behaviour;

5. *Maintenance:* The patient is continuing the new behaviour over an extended period of time

Key message

Always assess your client's stage of change.

Applying this to Bob

What stage of change are Bob and Dave currently at?

Any intervention will require the patient to adapt their behaviour in one way or another, be it taking time to attend a hospital appointment, adapting their diet or incorporating new exercise into their daily lives. In order to adhere to such advice, the person must be ready and prepared to accept this change. One way of assessing a patient's 'readiness' to change is to use the readiness ruler (see Figure 3.4). The readiness ruler can be used at the beginning of an intervention to help target the appropriate stage of change. Alternatively, it can be used during the intervention as a way of encouraging the patient to talk about reasons for change.

Thinking that change is important is not always enough for a person to move into the action phase. Sometimes a person is ready to make a change but is not confident that they are able to do so. For this reason, both readiness and confidence are addressed in motivation-based interventions.

The confidence ruler (see Figure 3.5) can be used to assess how confident patients are that they are able to adapt their behaviour, or it can be used as a hypothetical question to

On a scale of 1 to 10, how certain are you that you want to change this behaviour?

1	2	3	4	5	6	7	8	9	10
Not certain at all									Very certain
Pre-contemplation			Contemplation		Preparation			Action	

Figure 3.4 Readiness ruler

On a scale of 1 to 10, how confident are you that you can change this behaviour?

1	2	3	4	5	6	7	8	9	10

Not confident at all   Very confident

Figure 3.5 Confidence ruler

encourage patients to talk about how they would go about making a change. It is not necessary to actually show the patient a ruler, but it may be helpful, especially for young children or patients with low literacy and numeracy skills.

Based on the patient's confidence score, the healthcare professional might ask:

- You said your confidence was a 4, why not a 1 or a 2?
- Why not an 8 or a 9?
- What would it take to make it a 10?

The client's answers to these questions will tell you how resourceful they feel, as well as what potential barriers they have to conquer along the way. The final question will encourage the client to come up with their own solutions, tactics and ways to remove obstacles to change. It may also prove helpful to encourage the client to remember previous successes, to review obstacles and how they overcame them.

A person's belief in their ability to change is an important motivator (i.e. their self-efficacy). The healthcare professional can enhance a person's motivation to change by using open questions to elicit 'confidence talk'. Using negotiation and confidence building to persuade patients that they can change their behaviour is an important part of motivational interviewing.

Discussion point

Use the readiness and confidence rulers to assess your own motivation to change a specific aspect of your diet. For example, how important is it to you to eat more fruit and vegetables? On a scale of 1 to 10, how certain are you that you want to change this behaviour?

- What number did you choose?
- Why did you choose that number and not a lower/higher number?
- What would it take to make it a 10?

If you feel ready to change, now think about your confidence level. On a scale of 1 to 10, how confident are you that you can change this behaviour?

Make sure you pick a behaviour relevant to you. Now, how can you apply it to your client's diet?

Table 3.8 The ten processes of change

Process of change	What this means	Related to diet
Consciousness raising	Increasing information about self and problem: observations, confrontations, interpretations, bibliotherapy	Look for information on improving diet. Leaflets and information guidance
Self-re-evaluation	Assessing how one feels and thinks about oneself with respect to a problem: value clarification, imagery, corrective emotional experience	Feel disappointed with self when eating something unhealthy
Self-liberation	Choosing and commitment to act or belief in ability to change: decision-making therapy, New Year's resolutions, commitment-enhancing techniques	Making a decision to quit, and making a commitment to it
Counter-conditioning	Substituting alternatives for problem behaviours: relaxation, desensitisation, assertion, positive self-statements	Rather than grabbing a chocolate biscuit, have an apple or replace eating with a form of relaxation
Stimulus control	Avoiding or countering stimuli that elicit problem behaviours: restructuring one's environment (e.g. removing alcohol or fattening foods), avoiding high-risk cues, fading techniques	Remove fattening foods from the home. Replace with healthy foods
Reinforcement management	Rewarding oneself or being rewarded by others for making changes: contingency contracts, overt and covert reinforcement, self-reward	Make sure that friends and other members of the family provide reinforcement.
Helping relationships	Being open and trusting about problems with someone who cares: therapeutic alliance, social support, self-help groups	Weight watchers groups: social support from others
Dramatic relief	Experiencing and expressing feelings about one's problems and solutions: psychodrama, grieving losses, role playing	Emotional link between health and diet – worry and concern about their weight, or a recent health threat
Environmental re-evaluation	Assessing how one's problem affects the physical environment: empathy training, documentaries	How can the physical environment be improved by changing behaviour?
Social liberation	Increasing alternatives for non-problem behaviours available in society: advocating for rights of repressed, empowering, policy interventions	Wider adverts for healthy eating in society

Source: Based on Prochaska *et al.* (1988)

Processes of change

While stages of change represent dimensions that allow understanding of *when* changes occur, the processes of change (Prochaska *et al.*, 1988), outlined in Table 3.8, allow understanding of *how* changes occur. Ten processes of change have been identified, and specific processes are associated with particular stages of preparation for change. There is integration between the processes of change and the stages of change. Effective self-change depends on doing the right things (processes) at the right time (stages). With a mismatch in stage and processes, a successful behavioural change is unlikely to occur. Figure 3.5 highlights how these can be integrated when attempting to change an individual's diet.

Applying this to Bob

What process of change would you use for Bob and Dave?

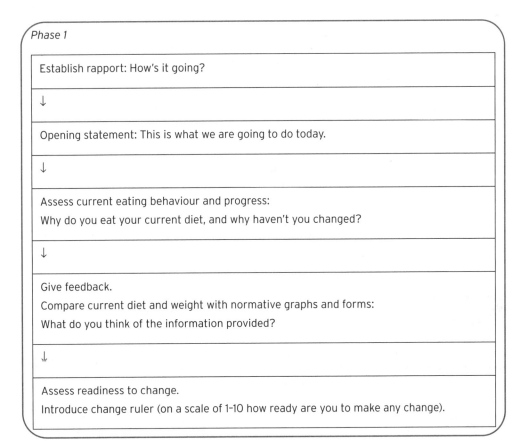

Figure 3.6 Changing diet through motivational interviewing

Phase 2

Tailor intervention approach		
↓	↓	↓
Stage 1	Stage 2	Stage 3
↓	↓	↓
Not ready	Unsure	Ready
↓	↓	↓
Goal: To raise awareness	Goal: To build motivation and confidence	Goal: To negotiate a plan
↓	↓	↓
Open-ended questions: 'What would need to be different for you to consider making new or additional changes in your diet?' Respect decisions Offer guidance	Explore ambivalence: 'What are the good and not so good things about making such changes?' Look to the future Refer to friends	Identify change option: 'What do you think you need to change?' Help set goals Develop action plans Summarise plan
	Close the encounter: Summarise the session Support self-efficacy	

Figure 3.6 continued

Conclusion

The consequences of a poor diet are more than just obesity. A poor diet can contribute to a range of illnesses, including coronary heart disease, cancer and type 2 diabetes. Conversely, eating the 'right' foods can prevent illness and promote health. Despite the wealth of evidence endorsing both the positive and negative impact diet can have on health, research suggests that many people do not eat a sufficiently healthy diet.

Several explanations have been put forward for why people eat what they do; these have ranged from the media, through to the social-environmental and the psychosocial. This chapter has also explored two key psychological models of eating behaviour: the developmental approach which emphasises the importance of learning and the development of food preferences, and the cognitive approach which explores the extent to which cognitions explain and predict behaviour.

Numerous interventions have been introduced to tackle the nation's poor diet; however, the effectiveness of such interventions remains poor. Future attempts to improve the nation's diet should be multi-component, include behaviour change strategies, provide ongoing support and, most importantly, be tailored to the needs of the individual; after all, one size does not fit all.

Putting this into action

Consider Bob's son Dave. How would you improve his diet using psychological principles? Also consider:

- how you would assess Dave's diet;
- how Dave's environment might influence his eating behaviour.

Summary points

- Diet can affect health through an individual's weight but also plays a role in the development of diseases such as CHD, cancer and diabetes.
- It is estimated that food-related ill-health is responsible for about 10% of morbidity and mortality in the UK.
- Healthy eating can be understood in terms of five major food groups and is important for promoting health and treating ill-health.
- Eating behaviour has been shown to be influenced by the media, the environment and social barriers such as availability, cost and time.
- The developmental approach emphasises the importance of learning and focuses on the development of food preferences in childhood. From this perspective, eating behaviour is influenced by exposure, social learning and associative learning.
- Research has demonstrated that self-efficacy, i.e. the belief in one's ability to exercise control over challenging demands, plays an important role in weight loss and weight maintenance.
- Decisional balance, or the individual's evaluation of the pros and cons, is a crucial component in the modification of dietary behaviours, as change is unlikely to occur until the reasons for change outweigh the reasons for staying the same.
- SMART goals are essential to diet improvement; that is, goals need to be Specific, Measrable, Achievable, Realistic and Timed.
- Motivational interviewing is a client-centred approach for eliciting behaviour change. It works by helping the patient to articulate why it is important for them to change while increasing their confidence that they are able to do so.

- According to the TTM, behaviour change can be thought of as a progression through a series of stages: pre-contemplation, contemplation, preparation, action and maintenance.
- Ten processes have been identified which explain how progression through the stages of change can occur. Effective self-change depends on doing the right things (processes) at the right time (stages).

Further resources

Conner, M. and Norman, P. (2007). *Predicting Health Behaviour,* 2nd edn. Berkshire: Open University Press.

Ogden, J. (2005). *The Psychology of Eating; From Healthy to Disordered Behaviour.* Oxford: Blackwell.

Thirlaway, K. and Upton, D. (2009). The *Psychology of Lifestyle: Promoting Healthy Behaviour.* London: Routledge.

Useful Web links

An online calculator for working out and interpreting a child's BMI is available at: www. healthforallchildren.co.uk on the parent's page.

Food Dudes healthy eating programme http://www.fooddudes.co.uk/

Eat well, be well – the Food Standards Agency website for consumer advice on healthy eating. It is packed with information and tips on eating a healthy balanced diet http://www. eatwell.gov.uk/

Cancer Prevention Research Centre provides a detailed overview of the Transtheoretical model, including the stages of change, processes of change, decisional balance and self-efficacy http://www.uri.edu/research/cprc/transtheoretical.htm

Motivational interviewing: resources for clinicians, researchers and trainers – provides background information on the practice of motivational interviewing http://www.motivational interview.org/

References

Ajzen, I. (1985). From intention to actions: A theory of planned behaviour. In J. Kuhl and J. Beckman (eds) *Action Control: From Cognition to Behaviour.* Available at: http:// www.people.umass.edu/aizen/publications.html (accessed 20 December 2007).

Bajekal, M., Primatesta, P. and Prior G. (2003). *Health Survey for England 2001.* London: The Stationery Office.

Bandura, A. (1986). *Social Foundations of Thought and Action: A Social Cognitive Theory.* Englewood Cliffs, NJ: Prentice-Hall.

Becker, M.H. and Rosenstock, I.M. (1984). Compliance with medical advice. In A. Steptoe and A. Mathews (eds) *Health Care and Human Behaviour.* London: Academic Press.

Birch, L. (1999). Development of food preferences. *Annual Review of Nutrition*, 19, 41–62.

Block, G., Patterson, B. and Subar, A. (1992). Fruit, vegetables and cancer prevention: A review of the epidemiological evidence. *Nutrition and* Cancer, 18, 1–29.

Boyce, T. (2007). The media and obesity. *Obesity Reviews*, 8 (1), 201–205.

Canoy, D. and Buchan, I. (2007). Challenges in obesity epidemiology. *Obesity Reviews*, 8(1), 1–11.

Connor Gorber, S., Tremblay, M., Moher, D. and Gorber, B. (2007). A comparison of direct vs. self-report measures for assessing height, weight and body mass index: A systematic review. *Obesity Reviews*, 8(4), 307–326.

Davis, A.M., Giles, A. and Rona, R. (2000). *Tackling Obesity: A Toolbox for Local Partnership Action*. London: Faculty of Public Health Medicine.

Dennis, K.E. and Goldberg, A.P. (1996). Weight control self-efficacy types and transitions affect weight-loss outcomes in obese women. *Addictive Behaviour*, 21, 103–116.

Department of Health. (1999). *Saving Lives: Our Healthier Nation*. London: The Stationery Office.

Department of Health. (2005). *Choosing a Better Diet: A Food and Health Action Plan*. London: TSO.

DePue, J.D., Clark, M.M., Ruggiero, L., Medeiros, M.L. and Pera, V. Jr. (1995). Maintenance of weight loss: A needs assessment. *Obesity Research*, 3, 241–248.

Doll, R. and Peto, R. (1981). *The Cause of Human Cancer*. Oxford: Oxford University Press.

Fishbein, M. and Ajzen, I. (1975). *Belief, Attitude, Intention and Behaviour. An Introduction to Theory and Research*. Available at: http://www.people.umass.edu/aizen/publications.html (accessed 20 December 2007).

Food Dude Healthy Eating Programme (2006). *The Food Dudes 1 page summary*. Available at: http://www.fooddudes.co.uk/documents/one_page_summary.pdf (accessed 22 December 2007)

Food Standards Agency (2004). Defusing the diet time bomb. Food and Beverage Conference, Queen Elizabeth Conference Centre. London: FSA.

Food Standards Agency (FSA) (2008). The eatwell plate. Available at: http://www.eatwell. gov.uk/healthydiet/eighttipssection/8tips (accessed 2 April 2008).

French, S.A., Perry, C.L., Leon, G.R. and Faulkerson, J.A. (1996). Self-esteem and change in body mass index over 3 years in a cohort of adolescents. *Obesity Research*, 4(1), 27–33.

Gratton, L., Povey, R. and Clark-Carter, D. (2007). Promoting children's fruit and vegetable consumption: Interventions using the Theory of Planned Behaviour as a framework. *British Journal of Health Psychology*, 12(4), 639–650.

Hancox, R.J. and Poulton, R. (2006). Watching television is associated with childhood obesity: But is it clinically important? *International Journal of Obesity*, 30, 171–175.

Haslam, D. and James, W.P. (2005). Obesity. *Lancet*, 366, 1197–1209.

Henderson, L., Gregory, J. and Swan, G. (2002). *The National Diet and Nutrition Survey, Volume 1; Adults aged 19 to 64 years. Types and Quantities of Foods Consumed*. Available at: http://www.food.gov.uk/multimedia/pdfs/ndnsprintedreport.pdf (accessed 3 December 2007).

Horne, P.J., Tapper, K., Lowe, C.F., Hardman, C.A., Jackson, M.C. and Woolner, J. (2004). Increasing children's fruit and vegetable consumption; a peer modelling rewards-based intervention. *European Journal of Clinical Nutrition*, 58, 1649–1660.

Janis, I.L. and Mann, L. (1977). *Decision Making: A Psychological Analysis of Conflict, Choice and Commitment.* New York: Free Press.

Jeffery, R.W., Bjornson-Benson, W.M., Rosenthal, B.S., Lindquist, R.A., Kurth, C.L. and Johnson, S.L. (1984). Correlates of weight loss and its maintenance over two years of follow-up among middle aged men. *Preventive Medicine,* 13, 155-168.

Kearney, M., Bradbury, C., Ellahi, B., Hodgson, M. and Thurston, M. (2005). Mainstreaming prevention: Prescribing fruit and vegetables as a brief intervention in primary care. *Journal of the Royal Institute of Public Health,* 119, 981-986.

Lowe, C.F., Horne, P.J., Bowdery, M.A., Egerton, C. and Tapper, K. (2001). Increasing children's consumption of fruit and vegetables. *Public Health Nutrition,* 4(2a), 387.

Lowe, C.F., Horne, P.J. and Hardman, C.A. (2007). *Changing the Nation's Diet: A Programme to Increase Children's Consumption of Fruit and Vegetables: Working Paper No. 5.* Available at: http://www.fooddudes.co.uk/documents/Working_paper_no5.pdf (accessed 11 December 2007).

Lowe, C.F., Horne, P.J., Tapper, K., Jackson, M., Hardman, C.A., Woolner, J., Bowdery, M.A. and Egerton, C. (2002). *Changing the Nation's Diet: A Programme to Increase Children's Consumption of Fruit and Vegetables.* End of project report. Bangor: University of Wales.

McPherson, K., Marsh, T. and Brown, M. (2007). *Foresight Tackling Obesities: Future Choices – Modelling Future Trends in Obesity and Their Impact on Health.* London: Department of Innovation, Universities and Skills.

National Audit Office. (2001). *Tackling obesity in England.* London: The Stationery Office.

National Institute for Health and Clinical Excellence (NICE). (2006). *Obesity: Guidance on the Prevention, Identification, Assessment and Management of Overweight and Obesity in Adults and Children.* Available at: http://www.nice.org.uk/nicemedia/pdf/word/CG43NICE Guideline.doc (accessed 11 December 2007).

National Institute for Health and Clinical Excellence (NICE) (2007). *Behaviour Change at Population, Community and Individual Levels.* Available at: http://www.nice.org.uk/ nicemedia/pdf/PH006guidance.pdf (accessed 9 July 2007).

Ness, A.R. and Powles, J.W. (1997). Fruit and vegetables and cardiovascular disease: A review. *International Journal of Epidemiology,* 26, 1-13.

Ofcom. (2004). *Childhood Obesity: Food Advertising in Context.* Available at: http://www. ofcom.or.uk/research/tv/reports/food_ads/report.pdf (accessed 20 December 2007).

Ofcom. (2006). *Annex 7 – Impact Assessment Consultation on Television Advertising of Food and Drink to Children.* Joint FSA/DoH Analysis; 2. London: Ofcom.

Prochaska, J.O. and DiClemente, C.C. (1983). Stages and processes of self-change smoking: Towards and integrative model of change. *Journal of Consulting and Clinical Psychology,* 51, 390-395.

Prochaska, J. O., DiClemente, C.C. and Norcross, J. C. (1992). In search of how people change: Application to addictive behaviors. *American Psychologist,* 47(9), 1102-1114.

Prochaska, J.O., Velicer, W.F., DiClemente, C.C. and Fava, J. (1988). Measuring processes of change: Applications to the cessation of smoking. *Journal of Consulting and Clinical Psychology,* 56, 520-528.

Rayner, M. and Scarborough, P. (2005). The burden of food related ill health in the UK. *Journal of Epidemiology and Community Health,* 59, 1054-1057.

Robinson, T.N. (1999). Reducing children's television viewing to prevent obesity: A random-ized controlled trial. *Journal of American Medical Association*, 282(16), 1561-1567.

Rodin, J., Elias, M., Silberstein, L.R. and Wagner, A. (1988). Combined behavioural and phar-macologic treatment for obesity: Predictors of successful weight maintenance. *Journal of Consulting and Clinical Psychology*, 56, 399-404.

Rogers, R.W. (1985). Attitude change and information integration in fear appeals. *Psychological Reports*, 56, 179-182.

Schwarzer, R. (1992). Self-efficacy in the adoption and maintenance of health behaviours: Theoretical approaches and a new model. In R. Schwarzer (ed) *Self-efficacy: Thought Control of Action*. Washington, DC: Hemisphere.

Strategy Unit. (2008). *Food: An Analysis of the Issues*. Available at: http://www.cabinetoffice.gov.uk/strategy/~/media/assets/www.cabinetoffice.gov.uk/strategy/food/food_analysis%20pdf.ashx (accessed 15 July 2008).

Stroebe, W. and Stroebe, M.S. (1995). *Social Psychology and Health*. Suffolk: Open University Press.

Swinburn, B.A., Egger, G.J. and Raza, F. (1999) Dissecting obesogenic environments: The development and application of a framework for identifying and prioritising environmental interventions for obesity. *Preventative Medicine*, 29, 563-570.

Unal, B., Critchley, J.A., and Capewell, S. (2004). Explaining the decline in coronary heart dis-ease mortality in England and Wales between 1981 and 2000. *Circulation*, 109, 1101-1107.

World Cancer Research Fund. (1997). *Food Nutrition, and the Prevention of Cancer: A Global Perspective*. Washington, DC: American Institute for Cancer Research.

World Health Organisation (WHO). (2004). *Report 916: Diet, Nutrition and the Prevention of Chronic Diseases*. Geneva: World Health Organisation.

Zaninotto, P., Wardle, H., Stamatakis, E., Mindell, J. and Head, J. (2006). *Forecasting Obesity to 2010*. Available at: http://www.dh.gov.uk/en/Piblicationsandstatistics/Publications/PublicationsStatistics/DH_4138630 (accessed 2 December 2007).

Chapter 4
Being active

LEARNING OBJECTIVES

At the end of this chapter you will:

- Understand what physical activity is and how to measure it
- Recognise how much physical activity is required to remain healthy
- Realise the current low levels of physical activity in the UK population
- Appreciate why some people do not achieve the recommended level of physical activity to remain healthy
- Have evaluated available interventions to help people increase their levels of physical activity

Case study

George is a 40-year-old manager of a large supermarket. He is responsible for the performance of his shop along with a number of staff. He works long hours since money is tight and commutes about 10 miles to and from work every day. George is married with three small children. His wife finds caring for three young children tiring and is very keen for George to get home promptly to help with the bedtime routine, although this is not always possible. They have only one car and it is needed in the evenings to take the older children to their various leisure activities. Whilst he enjoyed playing football at school, George stopped playing in his 20s due to a persistent knee injury. He has taken no exercise since, other than occasionally going swimming with his children.

Recently, George has been under a lot of pressure at work. He went to the GP reporting difficulty in sleeping and heart palpitations. After ensuring that George had no underlying severe physiological condition that was responsible for his symptoms, George's doctor diagnosed stress and depression and prescribed an anti-depressant together with beta blockers to control the heart palpitations.

George does not want to take either of the medications prescribed by the doctor. He comes to see you in your clinic to discuss alternative strategies to manage his symptoms. When he realises that exercise can be an effective treatment for stress and depression he is initially very enthusiastic about it but soon becomes despondent when he realises that it may mean him spending longer away from his wife and family. He feels that his wife will not support any activity that means he gets home any later and cannot see how he could incorporate an appropriate level of physical activity into his already busy day.

Discussion point

How would you work with George to build a sustainable physical activity routine that would help with his stress and depression?

Introduction

There are many opportunities for people to be physically active during the day, because physical activity in its broadest sense includes any movement. Formally, physical activity can be defined as:

Any bodily movement produced by the skeletal muscles that results in energy expenditure and is usually measured in kilocalories (kcal) per unit of time.
(Casperen et al., 1985, cited in Buckworth and Dishman, 2002, p. 28)

For many people in Western societies, including the UK, their normal daily occupations no longer require even moderate levels physical activity. The amount of non-leisure physical activity in the UK has declined consistently over the past few decades (Department of Health, 2004). Consequently, many health professionals find themselves attempting to encourage clients to increase the physical activity they do in their leisure-time through sport or exercise.

Applying this to George

George's occupation is mostly sedentary so any physical activity he achieves will be leisure-based or active transport.

Sport includes an element of competition that is not present in exercise activities. Biddle and Mutrie (1991, p. 8) define sport as:

Rule-governed, structured and competitive and involves gross motor movement characterised by physical strategy, prowess and chance.

The relationship between physical activity, exercise and sport can be conceptualised as a range of overlapping activities as illustrated in Figure 4.1.

At first, government strategies to increase physical activity in the population focused on encouraging more people to take up sport as a leisure-time activity: 'Sport for all' (www.olympic.org, accessed July 2009). However, more recently, the focus has moved away from sport towards exercise and then away from exercise towards occupational physical activity, because significant uptake of sport or exercise has not been achieved. Consequently, the emphasis of public health initiatives in the twenty-first century has been on encouraging individual, non-organised physical activity such as walking, cycling, gardening or housework. Sport and formal exercise have been losing credibility as potential sources of increased physical activity in the population. The current emphasis on physical activity and clear attempts to de-align physical activity from sport are evident in all public health documentation and policy (e.g. Department of Health 2003, 2004; Scottish Executive, 2005; Welsh Assembly Government, 2003; National Institute for Health and Clinical Excellence, 2006).

Key message

Recent attempts to increase physical activity have focused on exercise and non-organised physical activity such as gardening, walking or cycling rather than sport.

Nearly a decade after the Department of Health (1999) published their recommended physical activity levels of 30 minutes of moderate activity five times a week, and after 10

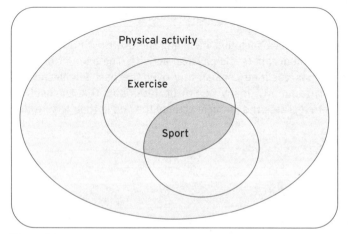

Figure 4.1 The relationship between physical activity, exercise and sport
Source: Thirlaway and Upton (2009), p. 87

Table 4.1 The percentages of men and women living in the UK achieving the government guidelines for weekly physical activity

Source of data	Percentage of people achieving government activity guidelines	Percentage of men achieving government activity guidelines	Percentage of women achieving government activity guidelines
Health Survey for England 2006 (Craig and Mindell, 2008)	34	40	28
Health Education Population Survey for Scotland 2005 (Gosling, 2006)	42	49	35
Welsh Health Survey 2008 (Welsh Assembly Government, 2009)	30	38	22
Northern Ireland Health and Social Wellbeing Survey 2005/2006 (Central Survey Unit, 2007)	30	33	28

years of policy and interventions attempting to encourage the population to meet these rec-ommendations, still only a third or less of the populations of England, Wales and Northern Ireland are meeting these criteria (Table 4.1). Scotland has the best figures and even here less than half of the population are physically active.

The impact of at least a decade of interventions to increase physical activity is not impres-sive (Table 4.1). The Health Survey for England (Primatesta, 2004) looked at trends in physi-cal activity between surveys carried out in 1997, 1998 and 2003. It did not find an overall trend for increasing activity, although it found some increases in the proportion of older people meeting the recommended activity levels. Other surveys of activity report similar findings. The Department of Health (2004) report that over the past two or three decades there has been a small increase in the proportion of people engaging in leisure activity but a reduction in routine physical activity, such as that achieved through necessary tasks of work, travel or running a home. The Office of National Statistics (2003) reported that distances walked annually dropped by 63 miles between 1975/6 and 2003. Similarly, distances cycled have dropped by 16 miles in the same period. The proportion of people who travel by walking or cycling has declined by 26% (Department of Health, 2004). Consequently, it has been argued that active transport could be a key factor in the achievement of healthy levels of physical activity (Jones et al., 2007).

Physical activity is currently the only lifestyle behaviour where men are more likely to achieve government guidelines than women (Table 4.1). Sport is often seen as a traditional male activity, which may contribute to this finding. Indeed, the Scottish Health Survey (Scottish Executive, 2005) asked about types of physical activity and found that the most common physical activity in men was sport/exercise whereas in women it was heavy housework.

Applying this to George

George would appear to follow a typical male trend of sports participation whilst young and a rapid decline into sedentary behaviour once middle-aged.

As both men and women get older their activity levels decline (Department of Health, 2003). The age-related decline in activity is more marked in men than women, but fewer women are active initially so by the time men and women are in their 60s their activities levels are similar. This supports the notion that men are achieving higher physical activity levels because they play more sport. Sporting participation decreases with age more markedly than any other physical activity (Scottish Executive, 2005). The relationship between physical activity and social class as measured by the National Statistics Socio-Economic Classification (NS-SEC) is complex and can be best described by an inverted U-shaped curve, with those at either end of the social class scale being the least likely to be active. The Health of Minority Ethnic Groups Survey (Joint Health Surveys Unit, 1999) measured participation in physical activity among the main minority groups in England. Compared to the general population, South Asian and Chinese men and women were much less likely to participate in physical activity of any kind. Bangladeshi men and women were the most inactive and were almost twice as likely as the general population to be classified as sedentary.

Key message

Only a minority of the population are achieving the government recommendations of physical activity. Physical activity is not consistent through the population and is influenced by sex, age, social class and ethnicity.

Government recommendations for physical activity

In the 1999 Department of Health document 'Saving Lives: Our Healthier Nation', the government recommended that adults took:

30 minutes of moderate exercise 5 times a week.
Department of Health (1999)

This has since been updated to read:

A total of at least 30 minutes a day of at least moderate intensity physical activity on 5 or more days of the week.
Department of Health (2004, p. 21)

The updated advice clearly indicates that the recommendations are for a minimum level of activity and that 'more is better'. A key issue here is the use of the word 'moderate'. What is moderate for one person may be either intense or light for the next. The American position on appropriate levels of physical activity is similar to that in the UK but attempts to address the problem of interpreting moderate by providing some examples of moderate physical activity:

Significant health benefits can be obtained by including a moderate amount of physical activity (e.g. 30 minutes of brisk walking or raking leaves, 15 minutes of running or 45 minutes of playing volleyball) on most, if not all, days of the week.
US Department of Health and Human Services (1999, p. 10)

The Department of Health (2004) also provide some useful guidance about what constitutes light, moderate and vigorous activity in their publication 'At least 5 a week' and their advice is summarised in Table 4.2.

The Department of Health (2004) recommend higher levels of physical activity for children:

At least 60 minutes of at least moderate intensity physical activity each day. At least twice a week this should include activities to improve bone strength (activities that pro-duce high physical stresses on the bones) muscle strength and flexibility.
Department of Health (2004, p. 21)

Table 4.2 Intensities and energy expenditure for common types of physical activity

Activity	Intensity	Energy expenditure (kcal equivalent of a person of 60 kg doing activity for 30 minutes)
Ironing	Light	69
Cleaning and dusting		75
Walking – strolling at 2 mph		75
Painting/decorating	Moderate	90
Walking – 3 mph		99
Vacuuming		105
Golf – walking and pulling clubs	Moderate	129
Badminton – social		135
Tennis – doubles		150
Walking – brisk 4 mph	Moderate	150
Mowing lawn – walking		165
Cycling – 10-12 mph		180
Aerobic dancing	Vigorous	195
Cycling – 12-14 mph		240
Swimming – slow crawl		240
Tennis – singles	Vigorous	240
Running – 6 mph (10 minutes/mile)		300
Running – 7 mph (8.5 minutes/mile)		345
Running – 8 mph (7.5 minutes/mile)		405

Source: Adapted from *At least 5 a day a week*, Department of Health (Department of Health 2004), © Crown Copyright 2004. Crown Copyright material is reproduced with permission under the terms of the Click-Use Licence

Applying this to George

How would George define his activity? What does the differing definitions of 'moderate' mean for the communication between practitioner and patient?

Both here and in the US the recommendations recognise that the appropriate level of physical activity for good health is not definitive. For weight loss there is clear evidence that higher levels of physical activity are necessary (Schoeller *et al.*, 1997). The Department of Health has responded by acknowledging that for obesity prevention between 45 and 60 minutes of at least moderate physical activity is probably necessary (Department of Health, 2004). Recently there have been strong calls in Britain for the advice to change from 'moderate' to 'vigorous', perhaps in recognition that a practitioner understanding of the term 'moderate' may be more vigorous than a lay understanding of it (BBC News, 2007). In America vigorous physical activity is now an integral aspect of the recommended physical activity levels (American College of Sports Medicine, 2007). The counterargument is that even small increases in physical activity can improve health (Church *et al.*, 2007) and setting more challenging targets may deter sedentary individuals from trying to take up physical activity. As is discussed in depth later in the chapter, and in Chapter 2, setting achievable goals is a cornerstone of effective behavioural change (Ajzen, 1998).

Key message

Any increase in physical activity improves health but the more active you are the better it is for your physical health.

Mental health

Whilst the government's physical activity recommendations are clearly aimed at improving physical health, there is increasing awareness and associated recommendations about the use of physical activity to improve psychological well-being (Crone *et al.*, 2009). It is acknowledged in a range of government policy documents that physical activity has a role in maintaining general well-being and also in the treatment of mental health problems. For example: 'At Least Five a Week' (Department of Health, 2004); 'Depression: Management of Depression in Primary and Secondary Care' (National Institute of Clinical Excellence, 2004); 'Making It Possible: Improving Mental Health and Well-being in England' (National Institute for Mental Health in England, 2005). It is not clear what is the best level of physical activity for well-being and/or treatment of mental health conditions but the current evidence suggests that lower levels of physical activity may improve psychological well-being than are required to improve physical health (Crone *et al.*, 2009). Indeed, some research suggests that overly vigorous physical activity, which participants feel is intense, may be detrimental to well-being.

Applying this to George

George is sedentary and looking to reduce his stress and depression. He is not currently obese. Setting him a goal of moderate physical activity should deliver the mental health benefits that he requires and may offer additional protective benefits against weight gain. Setting too hard a target may be unrealistic and potentially detrimental to self-efficacy.

Health consequences of low physical activity

If you are physically active you are likely to live longer than your sedentary colleagues regardless of whether you are young or old, male or female and regardless of ethnicity or social class (US Department of Health and Human Services, 1999; Pate *et al.*, 1995; Warburton *et al.*, 2006). Indeed, it has been suggested that adults who keep physically fit through activity are 50% less likely to die prematurely than sedentary adults (Warburton *et al.*, 2006). Others are more conservative in their estimates of benefits. The Department of Health (2004) have estimated that adults who are physically active have a 20–30% reduced risk of premature death.

Key message

Physical activity could reduce an individual's likelihood of premature death by 50%.

Physical activity influences a wide range of health conditions. For example, people who are physically active can achieve up to a 50% reduced risk of developing coronary heart disease, stroke, diabetes and some cancers (Department of Health, 2004). Physical activity can also play a role in reducing mental health problems such as depression, stress and anxiety (Crone *et al.*, 2009). Newly diagnosed individuals with such chronic diseases face not only a reduction in life expectancy but also a potential reduction in quality of life for the remainder of their lives. Whilst the relationship of physical activity to each disease is valuable, what makes physical activity particularly important is that it can prevent so many different diseases. Physical activity has an important role in treatment but it is its potential to prevent or delay disease onset that is so impressive and causes the Chief Medical Officer to conclude:

physical activity is one of the main contemporary public health issues.
Department of Health (2004)

Applying this to George

George has the dual problem of stress and depression so one benefit of utilising physical activity as a treatment option is that he can combat both of these conditions simultaneously, whereas the medical option involves two different types of medication. Furthermore, stress and depression, if untreated, are both related to weight gain and cardiovascular problems. Consequently, taking physical activity to relieve stress and depression will also serve a preventative function for George, reducing his risk of obesity, cardiovascular disease and type 2 diabetes.

Obesity

Levels of obesity are rising throughout the Western world and the UK is no exception to this trend. The Chief Medical Officer describes it as a new and serious threat to health because now nearly a quarter of the population are clinically obese. This reflects a threefold increase in obesity from 1980 to 2002 (Department of Health, 2004). Obesity is often associated with physical inactivity:

> *Obesity is the main visible sign of inactivity.*
> **Department of Health (2004, p. 20)**

Maintaining a healthy body weight should be easy. At its simplest, energy input simply has to equal energy output and weight will remain constant. If your energy intake exceeds your energy output, you will gain weight. Physical activity increases energy output and so decreases the likelihood that an individual will gain weight. However, moderate physical activity is unlikely to make a major contribution to weight loss. Physical activity, at the level suggested by the government, by itself can result in modest weight loss of around 0.5–1 kg a month (Pate *et al.*, 1995). Higher levels of physical activity can have more dramatic effects on body weight, but suggesting that obese individuals take even higher levels of physical activity than those recommended by the government is potentially dangerous and probably too challenging for currently sedentary individuals to achieve. Nevertheless, many health professionals and academics have called for new guidelines for weight-loss physical activity to be established. The Chief Medical Officer recognises this in his 2004 report, saying:

> *45–60 minutes of moderate activity per day may be needed to prevent the development of obesity . . . and people who have been obese and have managed to lose weight may need to do as much as 60–90 minutes activity a day in order to avoid regaining weight.*
> **Department of Health (2004, p. 5)**

Key message

The evidence suggests that for physical activity to have a significant effect on weight loss, 30 minutes of moderate activity on five days a week is unlikely to be a high enough level of activity. However, moderate levels of activity are more likely to protect individuals from excess weight gain.

Assessment of physical activity

It is beyond the scope of this text to provide a comprehensive review of all the available tools to measure physical activity – over 30 different measures have been reported – but there are a number of good textbooks where this can be obtained (Buckworth and Dishman, 2002; American College of Sports Medicine, 2005). To report the physical activity levels of different groups in the population you will need a measure that is quick and easy to administer to a large number of people. To measure physical activity as part of an individualised fitness programme, you might want a very detailed and accurate measure.

When you are thinking about measuring physical activity you need to consider whether you simply want to know the total time spent physically active in a given period or whether

Table 4.3 Categories of physical activity measurement

Method of measurement	Assessment	Information available
Measuring a physiological response to physical activity	Objective	Duration
		Intensity
Calculating the energy expenditure of physical activity	Objective	Duration
		Intensity
Assessing physiological adaptations to physical activity	Objective	Duration
		Intensity
Observing (either directly or indirectly) physical activity	Subjective	Duration
		Intensity
		Type
		Frequency

you wish to explore the physical activity in more depth. You may wish to know the time spent at different intensities of physical activity. You may wish to understand the impact that the physical activity is having on the physical state of an individual. You may wish to know the amount of energy a person is using, which might be particularly useful if you are interested in weight control or weight loss. You can measure levels of physical activity in one of four ways, described in Table 4.3.

Measures of physical activity can provide information about how often people exercise (frequency), how long they exercise (duration), how hard they work (intensity) and what type of activity (type) they choose to do (Table 4.3).

The first three methods are objective assessments of activity whereas observation is a more subjective assessment (Table 4.3). Objective measures of energy expenditure are more precise, giving reliable information about the duration and intensity of activity, but they can be costly and often not practical for large-scale studies. Furthermore, objective measures cannot tell you much about the type of activity undertaken and are seldom used longitudinally, so provide limited information about the frequency of physical activity The most usual form of observation is to use a questionnaire. The more complex questionnaires can provide detailed information about the type of activities undertaken and good information about duration and frequency but only imprecise information about the intensity of the activity (Table 4.3).

If you are going to use a questionnaire-based assessment of physical activity it is very important to use an established questionnaire that has been tested for reliability and validity. The best questionnaires will have been validated by an objective measure of physiological response to physical activity (such as heart-rate monitoring) or an objective measure of energy expenditure (such as doubly labelled water) (Krista and Casperen, 1997).

Discussion point

How would you measure physical activity in George? Would the different methods provide different results?

Why are people physically inactive?

The government guidelines for physical activity are not daunting and indeed many health professionals would like them to be more challenging, yet the majority of the population remain sedentary (American College of Sports Medicine, 2007). The reasons why are undoubtedly complex and not simply down to individual choices. In physical activity, perhaps more than any other lifestyle choice, the role of the physical environment is increasingly recognised as important (Jones *et al.*, 2007). Environmental, social, demographic, psychological and biological factors have all been implicated in physical activity and the relationship between these factors has been usefully conceptualised by Jones *et al.* (2007) as shown in Figure 4.2.

Obesogenic environments

Health promotion and education tend to be focused on the individual and persuading the individual to change, but the unsupportive nature of the modern environment is now recognised to play a role in the low levels of physical activity in Western societies. The term obesogenic has been adopted by policy makers and refers to an environment that is both supportive of high-calorie intake and unsupportive of physical activity (Foster *et al.*, 2006; Jones *et al.*, 2007).

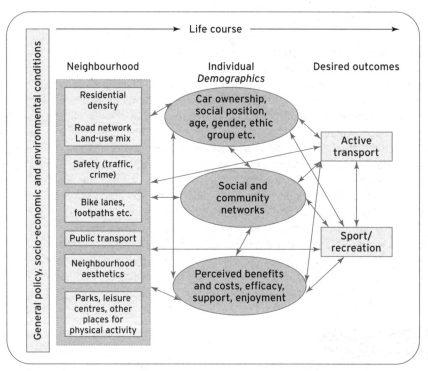

Figure 4.2 Evidence-informed model of the potential determinants of sport/physical activity
Source: Adapted from *Tackling obesities: future choices - obsofenic environments - evidence review,* Government Office for Science (Jones, A., Bentham., G. Foster, C., Hillsdon, M. and Panter, J. 2007), © Crown copyright 2007. Reproduced under the terms of the Click-Use Licence

So what is an obesogenic environment? It has not been clearly characterised, but certainly includes cultural, social and physical characteristics. Research on the impact of different environments on physical activity is beginning to emerge. A recent review of interventions that used the environment to encourage physical activity included 25 studies, 19 of which were studies aimed at encouraging the use of stairs (Foster et al., 2006). Whilst encouraging the use of stairs is undoubtedly a worthwhile venture, it is unlikely to increase the physical activity of any single individual by more than 10 minutes a day. The focus on encouraging stair use, often by decisional prompts, may reflect the difficulties with instigating more major changes to the environment. For instance, changing the environment to facilitate walking or cycling to work would probably require major changes. It might require the building of cycle paths and the provision of showers, lockers and bicycle sheds. Such major changes to the built environment, whilst sometimes undertaken, are seldom evaluated systematically to measure whether they encourage increased physical activity and, if so, in which population groups.

Whilst the physical environment is clearly a factor in physical activity and particularly in active transport, Jones et al. (2007) have concluded that the influence of the environment is probably small and the mechanisms are unclear. One thing is clear: the actual environment is less important than the way people perceive it. Jones et al. (2007) raise concerns that improving the environment by building more cycle paths, safe places to walk etc. may have its main effects on those who are already active rather than the sedentary. It doesn't matter how many cycle paths you build if people do not see themselves as able to use them. We need to understand why some people feel able to use good environmental resources to be physically active and some people do not. It is clear that interventions that both improve the environment and provide psychological support for change are more effective than a standalone change in the environment (National Institute for Health and Clinical Excellence, 2006).

Discussion point

How does the obesogenic environment influence George's physical activity behaviour? What in the environment could be changed to encourage an increase in his activity?

Psychological factors

Many different individual factors have been postulated to underpin physical activity behaviours; some of the key factors are presented in Table 4.4. The basic tenet of most health promotion campaigns is to present either the risk of an unhealthy behaviour and/or the benefits of a healthy behaviour. So health promotion is based on the assumption that individuals will weigh up the costs and benefits of physical activity and, based on that, make a decision about whether to take up physical activity. However, understanding that lack of physical activity is bad for your health has not been found to predict physical activity (Harrison et al., 2002). Indeed, there are studies that report no relationship between a perception of risk and physical activity (Blue, 2007).

The benefits of physical activity are also not related to engagement in sport or exercise (Rovniak et al., 2002). So it would appear that perceptions and beliefs about the health risks and benefits of physical activity and non-activity play only a small part in explaining variations in physical activity behaviours. Some authors have argued that they may be necessary

Table 4.4 Psychosocial factors implicated in behavioural change

Psychosocial factor	Potential to increase physical activity
Perception of the risk of physical inactivity	Minimal
Belief in the effectiveness of physical activity to improve health	Minimal
Objective barriers to physical activity	Minimal
Perceived behavioural control – perceived ability to overcome recognised barriers	Good
Social norms	Minimal as currently measured, but may be more useful if measured as perceived peer levels of activity
Self-efficacy	Good
Self-regulation	Good
Social support	Good

but are not sufficient to promote physical activity change. However, studies such as Blue (2007), which found no relationship between risk perception and activity levels, raise the question as to whether a perception of risk is necessary at all. It would seem that investing time or money in informing people about the costs of being sedentary and the benefits of being physically active is unlikely to generate widespread increases in physical activity.

Key message

People who understand that being sedentary is bad for their health and that being active is good for their health are still very likely to remain sedentary.

Barriers to performing physical activity, such as lack of access to resources or lack of time, have some relationship to whether people are active but perceived behavioural control over such barriers has been found to be a better predictor of physical activity than the actual barriers themselves (Conner and Norman, 2005). Individuals often cite a list of barriers to physical activity as an explanation for remaining sedentary. Working with them to look at how they can overcome these barriers and increase confidence in their own ability to control these external factors is more likely to generate change than changing the barriers. If barriers are removed, perhaps by improving leisure facilities in the local area, such strategies are more likely to be utilised if their implementation is supported by psychological support for uptake of the new behaviour.

Discussion point

How beneficial do you think the free swimming programmes available in certain parts of the country are? Or exercise prescriptions?

Key message

The physical environment is particularly relevant to physical activity as many activities are either performed outside or at a public venue such as a leisure centre. How people perceive their environment and the facilities available to them can influence whether they choose to be active.

Social norms refer to what is acceptable behaviour to the majority of an individual's peer group. Measures of social norms for physical activity consistently predict little if any variation in physical activity, indicating that social influences on intentions to exercise and exercise behaviour are less important than individual attributes (Hagger *et al.*, 2002; Godin and Kok, 1996). Some authors have argued that social norms are important but are difficult to measure, which is why there is no evidence that they influence the choices people make (Godin and Kok, 1996). The degree of social support that people have for them participating in exercise, rather than social norms, is a better predictor of whether people will exercise (Gruber, 2008; Rovnaik *et al.*, 2002). Despite the failure to demonstrate that social norms are a major factor in predicting variations in physical activity, Jones *et al.* (2007 p. 38), in their extensive review of obesogenic environments for the influential Foresight project, still conclude that 'capturing the concept of social norm and modifying that norm is one of the major public health challenges'.

There is evidence to suggest that social support plays an important role in adherence to physical activity programmes (McAuley *et al.*, 2000). For example, patients are more likely to adhere to an activity regime if their family are supportive (Oldridge, 1982). More recently, Bidonde *et al.* (2009) reported, in their study of older women, that group physical activity programmes can, in time, provide new social networks that support the participants not only in maintaining their physical activity but also, more extensively, in providing new friendships that can support individuals through challenges such as retirement and bereavement. Similarly, McAuley *et al.* (2000) have argued that exercise groups have a social structure and that interactions, friendships and alliances can form. Encouraging the development of social support within exercise groups could support adherence to exercise programmes but may provide the additional benefits of perceived well-being and life satisfaction that social support networks can bring.

Key message

Social support increases adherence to physical activity. Group exercise programmes, for example, can provide social support and increase the likelihood that people will stick to their exercise regime.

Applying this to George

George has a clear idea of what the benefits of activity would be for him. He lacks social support for taking up exercise and he perceives both the lack of support from his wife and his long working day as barriers to undertaking physical activity.

Probably, the most important psychological factor to emerge from research into physical activity behaviour is the concept of self-efficacy (Hagger *et al.*, 2002; Plotnikoff and Higgenbotham, 1998; Rovnaik *et al.*, 2002; Marshall and Biddle, 2001; Cox *et al.*, 2003). Self-efficacy refers to internal aspects of control such as perceived ability and self-confidence. University students who reported higher levels of exercise self-efficacy were more likely to be physically active (Rovniak *et al.*, 2002). Armstrong *et al.* (1993) and McAuley (1992) have reported that self-efficacy predicts both the adoption and maintenance of physical activity. Cox *et al.* (2003) found that self-efficacy for overcoming barriers was predictive of the adoption of physical activity and that increasing self-efficacy was critical to supporting positive changes in physical activity.

Self-efficacy has been argued to be enhanced by personal accomplishment or mastery, vicarious experience or verbal persuasion. According to the study by Strecher *et al.* (1995), people with high self-efficacy are more likely to utilise self-regulatory strategies, which in turn exerted a large total effect on physical activity in their study. Self-regulatory strategies include: goal setting, self-monitoring, planning and problem solving. Self-efficacy is not unrealistic optimism as it is based on experience, so in consequence realistic goals and plans that an individual can achieve are essential to increase self-efficacy (Luszczynska *et al.*, 2005). The importance of self-efficacy and self-regulation for effective interventions will be discussed later in the chapter.

Key message

Self-efficacy is the single most important factor in explaining physical activity behaviour and particularly in motivating change. People with high self-efficacy are more likely to be able to set achievable goals and overcome obstacles which in turn makes it more likely that they will persist in their physical activity.

Applying this to George

George has low self-efficacy about his ability to increase his physical activity. Helping him improve his self-efficacy will increase his chances of achieving his goals.

Stages of change

A key concept that has emerged from process models of change such as the Transtheoretical Model (TTM) is the idea that changing lifestyle behaviours is not a one-off decision but a continuous process and that people move between different motivational states (see Chapter 2). Identifying where individuals are in terms of stages of change may well result in more effective interventions to support the uptake of physical activity (Table 4.5).

Different types of psychological support are more likely to be effective at different stages. When individuals are in the pre-contemplation stage they may need education and motivational interventions to encourage them to move into the contemplation stage. Individuals who are contemplating or preparing to change may need to be helped to build self-efficacy

Table 4.5 The stages of change in relation to achieving the government recommendations for physical activity

Stages of change	Behavioural and motivational characteristics
Pre-contemplation	Individuals are sedentary and have no intention of doing 30 minutes of physical activity five times a week in the next six months
Contemplation	Individuals are sedentary but intend to take up physical activity to the level of the government recommendations within six months
Preparation	Individuals are taking some physical activity and intend to achieve acceptable levels of activity within six months
Action	Individuals have taken up physical activity and are exercising for at least 30 minutes five times each week. This is the least stable stage and relapse is likely
Maintenance	Individuals have been regular exercisers for six months or more and are unlikely to relapse

for the proposed change. Individuals who are in the action or maintenance stage will need support to stay motivated, again through increases in self-efficacy and in self-regulation. They need to ensure that their new physical activity behaviour becomes a habitual behaviour that they can maintain without constant cognitive effort.

Key message

Changing behaviour is not a one-off choice but an ongoing process.

Habitual behaviour

The powerful influence of past behaviour over future behaviour (Hagger et al., 2002; Connor and Norman, 2005) adds support to the argument that being physically active is an ongoing process. Consistent patterns of past behaviours are often referred to as habits. The reasons why people take up exercise may be different from the reasons why people maintain behaviour. Starting something new is a conscious choice but maintaining the behaviour may be habitual. Habits are those behaviours that we do automatically in response to a situation, rather than behaviours we think about. Past physical activity is an important predictor of future physical activity (Hagger et al., 2002; Connor and Norman, 2005), which suggests that developing physical activity habits is key to promoting long-term positive changes in physical activity. So what supports the development of a habit? Aarts et al. (1997) suggest that enjoyment is an essential aspect of habit formation. Traditional approaches to health behaviours have been negatively focused, looking predominantly at why people don't exercise. Consequently, enjoyment as a moderator of physical activity choices is seldom investigated. Nevertheless, studies that do consider affect report that individuals who are regular long-term exercisers report positive emotions during and following physical activity (Arent et al., 2000).

> **Key message**
>
> Many lifestyle behaviours, whilst initially conscious decisions, have become habitual.

Interventions to increase physical activity

Interventions to increase physical activity have been many and varied in many different settings with many different sections of society (Hillsdon et al., 2005; Kahn et al., 2002). Kahn et al. (2002) usefully differentiate between different interventions by categorising them as information-based, behavioural or environmental/policy-level interventions. Whilst many interventions will straddle these definitions, they do a least provide a starting point for evaluation (Table 4.6).

Information interventions

Information interventions can be as short and simple as point-of-decision prompts at the bottom of a building, where a choice of the lift or the stairs is available, or as complex as detailed individualised information given by a general practitioner (Hillsdon et al., 2005). Information can be provided through the media in written form or through radio and television campaigns. Increasingly, information is provided through the internet, such as the change4life campaign. In social cognitive terms an information intervention usually attempts to increase people's perception of risk from inactivity. Alternatively, or as well as, an information campaign may highlight the benefits of exercise for health. Most physical activity campaigns will take such a health-orientated focus, although reference to social benefits or enjoyment is not uncommon. Kahn et al. (2002) in their review of informational campaigns found no evidence that informational-only media-based campaigns were effective, which is what we would have predicted from the research evidence about communicating risk and benefits (Thirlaway and Upton, 2009). Similarly, Ogilvie et al. (2004) found no evidence that informational campaigns

Table 4.6 Physical activity interventions

Type of intervention	Aims
Information-based	To change knowledge and attitudes about the benefits and opportunities for physical activity within a community
Behavioural	To assist people in the development of behavioural management skills that enable them to adopt and maintain behavioural change and/or to create social environments that facilitate and enhance behavioural change
Environmental/policy	To change the structure of physical and organisational environments to provide safe, attractive and convenient places for physical activity

to increase active transport were successful. However, multi-component interventions, where media-based information plays a central part, are more likely to be successful at increasing physical activity (Kahn *et al.*, 2002; Brown *et al.*, 2006). Such multi-component campaigns usually include self-help groups and other forms of social support (Kahn *et al.*, 2002).

Decisional prompts at the base of buildings with a number of floors have been found to be effective in increasing the decision to take the stairs rather than the lift (Foster *et al.*, 2006), although whether these are truly informational interventions is arguable as they do not necessarily provide information but rather identify a healthy choice for an individual over which they have immediate control and minimal perceived or real barriers. Hillsdon *et al.* (2005) in their evidence briefing to the Health Development Agency reported that brief advice from a health professional supported by written materials was likely to produce modest short-term (12 weeks or less) increases in physical activity. Information given on an individual basis can be seen as directly relevant to the individual, who cannot ignore their own susceptibility as easily as they can information from media-based campaigns (see Box 4.1).

Box 4.1   Applying research in practice

An evaluation of an informational versus a motivational intervention (Hillsdon *et al.*, 2005)

This paper investigated the impact of two different communication styles in a primary health-care setting; 16,58 middle-aged men and women were assigned to a 30-minute intervention that was either:

1   a brief negotiation based on motivational interviewing techniques where clients were supported in coming to a decision about whether to attempt to increase their physical activity;

2   direct advice to take 30 minutes of physical activity five days a week in order to reduce the risks of inactivity;

3   no-intervention control group.

All participants were telephoned regularly following the initial 30-minute consultation, six times over a six-month period. The brief negotiation group were asked to report on their activities, whereas the direct advice group received more advice about the importance of physical activity.

Participants who received the brief negotiation intervention increased their physical activity more than the control participants. The brief negotiation group produced a greater reduction in diastolic blood pressure than the direct advice group.

Key message

Motivational interviewing techniques can be more effective than straightforward advice in promoting increased activity.

Applying this to George

Working with George in a client-centred way, using motivational interviewing techniques, is more likely to result in increased physical activity than giving him advice about the risks of inactivity and benefits of physical activity.

Behavioural interventions

Behavioural interventions are most likely to be at a small group or individual level of intervention and include strategies such as motivational interviewing and self-regulation. Hillsdon et al. (2005) concluded that interventions that taught behavioural skills and were tailored to individual needs were associated with more long-term changes than interventions without psychological intervention. Similarly, Kahn et al. (2002) found that individually adapted behavioural change programmes were effective in increasing physical activity levels. Further support for the value of psychologically based behavioural change programmes comes from Ogilvie et al. (2004), who found that targeted behavioural change programmes were the most effective way to promote walking and cycling. Behavioural change programmes work through a number of different psychological mechanisms. Firstly, they can provide regular contact with an exercise specialist who, seen regularly, will provide specific social support and perhaps also more general social support. Furthermore, an exercise specialist can set appropriate goals that foster and develop self-efficacy (Rovniak et al., 2002). Good behavioural change interventions include advice and help with goal setting, overcoming obstacles and developing social support, which facilitate uptake and maintenance of physical activity by increasing self-efficacy (Cox et al., 2003; Rovniak et al., 2002).

Motivational interviewing

Motivational interviewing (MI) is a technique first developed for use with dependent drinkers to encourage them to reduce their drinking. It has subsequently been adopted and adapted for use with a range of lifestyle behaviours. MI aims to increase an individual's motivation to consider change rather than showing them how to change. If a person doesn't want to change then it is irrelevant if they know how to do it or not. However, if a person is motivated to change then the interventions aimed at changing behaviour can begin. MI can therefore be viewed as the first stage of a process that moves people towards being physically active. The key aspects of MI are presented in Chapter 2. Motivational interviewing has not been used extensively with physical activity but it has been found to be more successful than simply advising people to be physically active (Box 4.1).

Key message

Motivational interviewing is a behavioural technique that encourages people to want to change.

Goal setting

The key to successful goal setting is setting challenging but realistic goals that enable people to feel they have achieved a goal and gives them confidence that they can achieve the next sub-goal on their way to a healthy level of physical activity (Chapter 2; Table 4.7). Getting goals right is a tricky task and requires understanding the physical capacities of an individual, their level of skill and their self-efficacy for the various activities that may be involved. Consequently, it requires the skilled input of a health or exercise specialist. It is not enough to set appropriate individualised goals – individuals need to get regular feedback, which may be provided by the health professional or alternatively it may be possible for an individual to self-monitor performance and receive feedback in that way. The key strategies for successful goal setting in relation to physical activity are presented in Table 4.7.

Key message

The key to successful goal setting is setting challenging but realistic goals.

Table 4.7 Effective strategies in goal setting to increase physical activity

Strategy	Example
Explore client motivation. This might be done using the stages of change paradigm. Pre-contemplation clients are not ready for goal setting	A middle-aged women refers herself to you to increase her physical activity levels to help her lose weight. Clearly, she is motivated to be more physically active. You need to explore the overarching goal. A weight loss goal may be less achievable than a stress reduction goal
Break down long-term goal into a series of short-term sub-goals and create an action plan	You might set the client a series of short-term goals, such as increasing weekly steps or getting off the bus two stops earlier to walk to work
Attempt where possible to set behavioural goals rather than physiological goals	If your client has an overarching aim of weight loss you should nevertheless encourage them to set behavioural goals rather than physiological 'pounds lost' targets
Evaluate client self-efficacy for the various behaviours involved in goal achievement	There are many different types of physical activity and the more confident the client is about performing an activity the more likely they are to achieve it
Tailor sub-goals to client to ensure they are challenging but realistic and perceived as such by the client	Your client may wish to set goals that are unrealistic; rapid weight loss is attractive to most individuals wishing to lose weight. You need negotiate a goal for which you are likely to be able to deliver positive feedback
Provide regular feedback to the client or provide a mechanism for the client to self-monitor performance and receive feedback	Feedback needs to be regular, supportive and reflect behavioural achievements and physiological achievements if appropriate
Goal adaptation	For long-term complex change the short-term sub-goals may need to be reviewed and renegotiated as the client's physiological status and self-efficacy change in response to behavioural adaptation

It has been argued that setting behavioural goals, such as attending an exercise class, rather than physiological goals, such as weight loss, are more effective goals to set because the individual has more direct control over behaviour. Furthermore, Segar *et al.* (2008) found that middle-aged women who had weight loss goals participated in less physical activity than their contemporaries who had physical activity goals focused on well-being and stress reduction. It may be sensible when working with people who wish to lose weight to encourage them to set interim goals around well-being in order for them to achieve the physical activity levels that they require.

Applying this to George

To increase George's self-efficacy about his ability to be more active, he needs to be encouraged to set himself challenging but achievable goals that he can review regularly.

Pedometers

One thing that has emerged from work on goal setting and physical activity is that positive feedback about the successful achievement of goals is key to continued success (Nigg *et al.*, 2008). Regular professional feedback requires significant input from a health professional, so the possibility of feedback through self-monitoring using a relatively cheap monitoring system such as a pedometer has generated a lot of interest. Pedometers have recently become commonplace and the target of 10,000 steps a day is well known (Slack, 2006; Bennett *et al.*, 2006). Research has demonstrated that pedometers can be used successfully as part of a goal-setting programme to increase both the number of steps taken daily (Normand, 2008) and the pace at which individuals walk (Johnson *et al.*, 2006). However, the problem of setting goals that are both challenging and realistic remains, and the general goal of 10,000 steps a day would appear to have been too challenging for many individuals and resulted in failure to meet the daily target, loss of self-efficacy and giving up on the walking programme. The conclusion of the National Institute for Health and Clinical Excellence (NICE, 2006) is that there is no evidence that the general use of pedometers increases physical activity levels either in the long or short term. The moderately successful 10,000 steps Rockhampton Project (Brown *et al.*, 2006) did demonstrate modest increases in physical activity in their community but only in women (Box 4.2).

Box 4.2   Applying research in practice

10,000 Steps Rockhampton Project (Brown et al., 2006)

This community-wide project attempted to change the physical activity of a whole community by a complex set of interventions at multiple levels. It included a range of intervention strategies:

● pedometers as self-monitoring and goal-setting instruments;

● two overarching goals: 10,000 steps a day and Every Step Counts;

● social marketing using print, radio and TV;

→

- promotion of physical activity by health professionals;
- environmental support, improvements to footpaths etc.

This ambitious study found that women were the early adopters of the project and that over the 18 months of the project women's activity levels increased, with a 5% increase in women who could be categorised as 'sufficiently active'. The authors of the review of the project acknowledge that this is a modest increase in activity but, given the population of 60,000, it is still about 3,000 women who increased their physical activity to some degree. It is not clear why the intervention was more successful with women and this is something that would need further exploration before embarking on similar projects.

Key message

Multi-level community-based interventions can be successful but are hard to evaluate.

Social support

Goal setting, as described previously, requires sustained input from a health or exercise specialist. One advantage of this is that the professional can provide specific social support for physical activity. The feedback that they provide is a form of social support for the attempted change in behaviour. Such behavioural-specific social support has also been demonstrated to support physical activity when provided by friends and peers (Jeffery and French, 1996). Exercise groups can also provide social support for maintaining physical activity (Gruber, 2008). Furthermore, there is evidence from older women that exercise groups can develop over time to provide not only specific social support for maintaining physical activity, but also more general emotional support as the relationships made within the group develop (Bidonde et al., 2009). Consequently, encouraging individuals to participate in exercise groups has the potential to benefit health both through the increased levels of physical activity and also through the social support networks that individuals may develop over time.

Discussion point

George's social support network is mainly based on his family. Will their general emotional support provide the support for his proposed change in physical activity or will he require further specific social support?

Exercise referral schemes

Exercise referral schemes are very popular in the UK, with an estimated 600 schemes currently running. These schemes have the opportunity to provide many of the psychological support strategies described earlier, such as social support and goal setting which are known to promote physical activity. However, The National Institute for Health and Clinical

Excellence (2006) report that there is no evidence that such schemes successfully increase physical activity levels in the long term. Two trials suggested that exercise referral schemes were effective in the short term (6 to 12 weeks) but four studies reported no increase in physical activity over the longer term (12 weeks to one year). A more theoretical approach to exercise referral, with appropriate psychological training of exercise providers, may improve the outcomes from this widespread and major intervention. In 2006 the National Institute for Health and Clinical Excellence recommended that exercise referral schemes should be properly evaluated and this process is currently being undertaken.

Environmental interventions

Public health policy is focusing on the obesogenic environment and integrated health and transport strategies to promote active transport (Ogilvie et al., 2004; Foster et al., 2006; Jones et al., 2007). Currently, the evidence is that the various active transport schemes have not resulted in more active transport (Office of National Statistics, 2003). However, the impact of major environmental changes, such as the building of cycle paths, takes time to impact on the behaviour of individuals. It is plausible that we will see a reversal of the decline in active transport over the next decade. The evidence indicates that perception of the environment is more important than the environment per se (Jones et al., 2007). Consequently, environmental adaptations will need to be supported by behavioural interventions to support adaptation to the environment and positive changes in physical activity, or we run the risk of supporting only the physical activity behaviours of the currently active (Jones et al., 2007). One way forward is to adopt a whole community approach such as that carried out in Rockhampton, Australia in 2002/2003. This project attempted to address informational, psychological and environmental factors simultaneously (see Box 4.2).

Conclusion

Educational campaigns to increase physical activity have had little impact on population levels of physical activity. We live in an obesogenic environment which discourages physical activity. People need psychological support to enable them to become more physically active and this support will need to be long term if they are both to adopt and maintain healthy levels of physical activity. Currently, evidence suggests that self-regulation through goal setting, self-monitoring and feedback is the most effective way to promote physical activity. Well-set goals can build self-efficacy and support physical activity in the long term. It is clear that enjoyment is central to the long-term maintenance of physical activity but it is not clear why some people enjoy physical activity and others do not. This is an area worthy of further research.

Putting this into action

George is one of the majority of people who understands that physical activity would improve his health and he would like to be more active but he cannot see how he can overcome the barriers he perceives to being more physically active. He doesn't need any more

→

information about his risk or the benefits of physical activity. He needs support in finding a solution that is appropriate to his personal situation. He needs to be encouraged to make small changes to his activity that will give him a sense of achievement and the self-efficacy to attempt further changes. If he wishes to utilise active transport as a strategy he will need to understand the habitual nature of activities such as driving to work and attempt to break the bad habit of driving to work and establish the good habit of cycling to work. He will lack social support for physical activity if it reduces his time in the home, so utilising active transport will minimise the impact of increasing his physical activity on his family and increase the likelihood that his wife will be supportive. Furthermore, if cycling to work means the car is more available to his wife she may be more supportive.

Summary points

- Only a minority of the population achieve the government recommendations for physical activity.
- Women are less likely to be active than men at first, but activity by men declines dramatically during the lifespan so that by the time people are in their 60s activity levels are similar in the two sexes.
- What makes physical activity so important for health outcomes is the strength of its effect over such a wide range of conditions.
- People generally understand the risks of being sedentary and the benefits of physical activity but still do not get active.
- Self-efficacy is the best predictor of successful increases of physical activity.
- The establishment of good physical activity habits may be crucial in the promotion of physical activity.
- Perceptions of the environment may be more important than the objective environment for physical activity.

Further resources

Dugdill, L., Crone, D. and Murphy, R. (2009). *Physical Activity and Health Promotion*. Oxford: Wiley-Blackwell.

Useful Web links

Change for life 0300 123 4567 http://www.nhs.uk/Change4Life
British Heart Foundation http://www.bhfactive.org.uk
Diabetes UK http://www.diabetes.org.uk

References

Aarts, H., Paulussen, T. and Schaalma, H. (1997). Physical exercise habit: On the conceptualization and formation of habitual health behaviours. *Health Education Research*, 21, 363-374.

Ajzen, I. (1998). Models of human social behaviour and their application to health psychology. *Psychology and Health*, 13, 735-739.

American College of Sports Medicine. (2005). *ACSM's guidelines for Exercise Testing and Prescription*. Philadelphia, PA: Lippincott, Williams & Wilkins.

American College of Sports Medicine. (2007). *Updated Physical Activity Guidelines*. Available at: www.acsm.org (accessed September 2007).

Arent, S.M., Landers, D.M. and Etrier, J.L. (2000). The effects of exercise on mood in older adults: A meta-analysis review. *Journal of Aging and Physical Activity*, 8, 407-430.

Armstrong, C., Sallis, J., Hovell, M. and Hofstetter, C.R. (1993). Stages of change, self-efficacy and the adoption of vigorous exercise: A prospective analysis. *Journal of Sport and Exercise Psychology*, 15, 390-402.

BBC News. (2007). Exercise 'must be tough to work'. To be healthy, you really do need to break into a sweat when you exercise, say experts. Available at: www.bbc.co.uk (accessed September 2007).

Bennett, G.G., Wolin, K.Y., Viswanath, K., Askew, S. Puleo, E. and Emmons, K.M. (2006). Television viewing and pedometer-determined physical activity amoung multi-ethnic residents of low income housing. *American Journal of Public Health*, 96, 1681-1685.

Biddle, S. and Mutrie, N. (1991). *Psychology of Physical Activity and Exercise*. London: Springer-Verlag.

Bidonde, J.M., Goodwin, D.L. and Drinkwater, D.T. (2009). Older women's experiences of a fitness program: The importance of social networks. *Journal of Applied Sport Psychology*, 21(1), S86-S101.

Blue, C.L. (2007). Does the theory of planned behaviour identify diabetes-related cognitions for intention to be physical active and eat a healthy diet? *Public Health Nursing*, 24(2), 141-150.

Brown, W.J., Mumery, K., Eakin, E. and Schofield, G. (2006). 10,000 steps Rockhampton: Evaluation of a whole community approach to improving population levels of physical activity. *Journal of Physical Activity & Health*, 3, 1-14.

Buckworth, J. and Dishman, R. (2002). *Exercise Psychology*. London: Human Kinetics.

Central Survey Unit. (2007). *Northern Ireland Health and Social Well-Being Survey 2005/6*. Belfast: Central Survey Unit.

Church, I.S., Earnest, C.P., Skinner, J.S. and Blair, S.N. (2007). Effects of different doses of physical activity on cardiorespiratory fitness among sedentary overweight or obese post menopausal women with elevated blood pressure: A randomised controlled trial. *Journal of American Medical Association*, 297, 2081-2091.

Conner, M. and Norman, P. (2005). *Predicting Health Behaviour*, 2nd edn. Berkshire: Open University Press.

Cox, K.L., Gorely, T.J., Puddey, I.B. and Beiline, L.J. (2003). Exercise behaviour change in 40 to 65-year old women: The SWEAT Study (Sedentary Women Exercise Adherence Trial). *British Journal of Health Psychology*, 8, 477-495.

Craig, R. and Mindell, J. (2008). *Health Survey for England 2006. Volume 1: Cardiovascular Disease and Risk Factors in Adults*. London: The Information Centre.

Crone, D., Heaney, L. and Owens, C.S. (2009). Physical activity and mental health. In L. Dugdill, D. Crone and R. Murphy (eds). Physical Activity and Health Promotion. London: Wiley-Blackwell.

Department of Health. (1999). *Saving Lives: Our Healthier Nation*. London: The Stationery Office.

Department of Health. (2003). *Health Survey for England*. London: HMSO.

Department of Health (2004). At Least Five a Week. London: Department of Health.

Foster, C., Hillsdon, M., Cavill, N., Bull, F., Buxton, K. and Crombie, H. (2006). *Interventions that Use the Environment to Encourage Physical Activity: Evidence Review*. London: NICE.

Godin, G. and Kok, G. (1996). The theory of planned behaviour: A review of its applications to health-related behaviours. *American Journal of Health Promotion*, 11, 87-98.

Gosling, R. (2006). *Health Education Population Survey: Update from 2005 Survey*. Edinburgh. NHS Health Scotland.

Gruber, K.J. (2008). Social support for exercise and dietary habits among college students. *Adolescence*, 43(171), 557-575.

Hagger, M.S., Chatzisarantis, N.L.D. and Biddle, S.J.H. (2002). A meta-analytic review of the theories of reasoned action and planned behaviour in physical activity: Predictive validity and the contribution of additional variables. *Journal of Sport and Exercise Psychology*, 24, 3-32.

Harrison, J.A., Mullen, P.D. and Green, L.W. (2002). A meta-analysis of studies of the health belief model with adults. *Health Education Research*, 7, 107-116.

Hillsdon, M., Foster, C., Cavill, N., Crombie, H. and Naidoo, B. (2005). *The Effectiveness of Public Health Interventions for Increasing Physical Activity among Adults: A Review of Reviews*, 2nd edn. London: Health Development Agency.

Jeffery, R.W. and French, S.A. (1996). Socioeconomic status and weight control practices among 20 to 45 year old women. *American Journal of Public Health*, 86(7), 1005-1010.

Johnson, S.T., McCargar, L.J., Bell, G.J., Tudor-Locke, C., Harber, V.J. and Bell, R.C. (2006). Distilling a complex prescription for type 2 diabetes management through pedometry. *Diabetes Care*, 29(7), 1654-1655.

Joint Health Surveys Unit. (1999). *Health Survey for England: Health of Minority Ethnic Groups 1999*. London: The Stationery Office.

Jones, A., Bentham, G., Foster, C., Hillsdon, M. and Panter, J. (2007). *Tackling Obesities: Future Choices – Obesogenic Environments – Evidence Review*. London: United Kingdom Government Foresight Programme, Office of Science and Innovation.

Kahn, E., Ramsey, L., Brownson, R., Heath, G., Howze, E., Powell, K., Stone, E., Rajab, M., Corso, P. and the Task Force on Community Preventive Services. (2002). The effectiveness of interventions to increase physical activity: A systematic review. *American Journal of Preventative Medicine*, 22, 73-107.

Krista, A.M. and Casperen, C.J. (1997). Introduction to a collection of physical activity questionnaires. *Medicine and Science in Sports and Exercise*, 29(6), supplement 5-9.

Luszczynska, A., Mohamed, N.E. and Schwarzer, R. (2005). Self efficacy and social support predict benefitingfinding 12 months after cancer surgery. The mediating role of coping strategies. *Psychology, Health and Medicine*, 10, 365-366.

Marshall, S.J. and Biddle, S.J.H. (2001). The transtheoretical model of behavior change: A meta-analysis of applications to physical activity and exercise. *Annals of Behavioral Medicine*, 23, 229-46.

McAuley, E. (1992). The role of efficacy cognitions in the prediction of exercise behaviour in middle-aged adults. *Journal of Behavioural Medicine*, 15, 65-88.

McAuley E., Blissmer, B., Marquez, D.X., Jerome, G.J., Kramer, A.F. and Katula, J. (2000). Social relations, physical activity and well-being in older adults. *Preventive Medicine*, 31, 608-617.

National Institute for Health and Clinical Excellence. (2004). *Depression: Management of Depression in Primary and Secondary Care*. London: NICE.

National Institute for Health and Clinical Excellence. (2006). *Public Health Intervention Guidance no. 2. Four commonly used methods to increase physical activity: brief interventions in primary care, exercise referral schemes, pedometers and community-based exercise programmes for walking and cycling*. London: NICE.

National Institute for Mental Health in England. (2005). *Making It Possible: Improving Mental Health and Well-being in England*. Leeds: NIMHE.

Nigg, C.R., Borrelli, B., Maddock, J. and Dishman, R.K. (2008). A theory of physical activity maintenance. *Applied Psychology: An international review*, 57(4), 544-560.

Normand, M.P. (2008). Increasing physical activity through self-monitoring, goal setting and feedback. *Behavioural Interventions*, 23, 227-236.

Office of National Statistics. (2003). *National Travel Survey: 2003 Final Results*. London: The Stationery Office.

Ogilvie, D., Egan, M., Hamilton, V. and Pettricrew, M. (2004). Promoting walking and cycling as an alternative to using cars: Systematic review. *British Medical Journal Online*, BMJ,doi:10.1136/bmj.38216.714560.55

Oldridge, N.B. (1982). Compliance and exercise in primary and secondary prevention of coronary heart disease: A review. *Preventive Medicine*, 11(1), 56-70.

Pate, R.R., Pratt, M., Blair, S.N., Haskell, W.L., Macera, C.A., Bouchard, C., Buchner, D., Ettinger, W., Heath, G.W., King, A.C., Kriska, A., Leon, A.S., Marcus, B.H., Morris, J., Paffenbarger, R.S., Patrick, K., Pollock, M.L., Rippe, J.M., Sallis, J. and Wilmore, J.H. (1995). Physical activity and public health - a recommendation from the Centers for Disease Control and Prevention and the American College of Sports Medicine. *Journal of the American Medical Association*, 273, 402-407.

Plotnikoff, R.C. and Higginbottom, N. (1998). Protection motivation theory and the prediction of exercise and low-fat diet behaviours among Australian cardiac patients. *Psychology and Health*, 13, 411-429.

Primatesta, P. (2004). *Health Survey for England 2004 - Updating of Trend Tables to Include 2005 Data*. London: The Stationery Office.

Rovniak, L.S., Anderson, E.S., Winett, R.A. and Stephens, R.S. (2002). Social cognitive determinants of physical activity in young adults: A prospective structural equation analysis. *Annals of Behavioural Medicine*, 24, 149-156.

Schoeller, D.A., Shay, K. and Kushner, R. (1997). How much physical activity is needed to minimize weight gain in previously obese women? *American Journal of Clinical Nutrition*, 66, 551-556.

Scottish Executive. (2005). *The Scottish Health Survey 2003*. Edinburgh: Scottish Executive.

Segar, M.L., Eccles, J.S. and Richardson, C.R. (2008). Type of physical acitivy goal influences participation in healthy midlife women. *Women's Health Issues,* 18, 281-291.

Slack, M.K. (2006). Interpreting current physical activity guidelines and incorporating them into practice for health promotion and disease prevention. *American Journal of Health System Pharmacy,* 63, 1647-1653.

Sport for all. www.olympic.org (accessed July 2009).

Strecher, V.J., Seijts, G.H., Kok, G.J., Latham, G.P., Glasgow, R., DeVellis, B., Meertens, R.M. and Bulger, D.W. (1995). Goal setting as a strategy for health behaviour change. *Health Education Quarterly* 22(2) 190-200.

Thirlaway, K.J. and Upton, D. (2009). *The Psychology of Lifestyle: Promoting Healthy Behaviour*. London. Routledge

US Department of Health and Human Services. (1999). *Physical Activity and Health: A Report of the Surgeon General*. Atlanta, GA: Us Department of Health and Human Services, Centres for Disease Control and Prevention, National Center for Chronic Disease Prevention and Health Promotion.

Warburton, D.E.R, Whitney, N.C. and Bredin, S.S.D. (2006). Health benefits of physical activity: The evidence. *Canadian Medical Association Journal,* 174, 801-809.

Welsh Assembly Government. (2009). *Welsh Health Survey 2008: Initial Headline Results*. Cardiff: Welsh Assembly Government.

Chapter 5
Sensible drinking

LEARNING OBJECTIVES

At the end of this chapter you will:

- Have recognised the extent of harmful and binge drinking in the UK
- Understand the government recommendations for sensible drinking
- Have reviewed the health and economic consequences of drinking alcohol
- Have evaluated the role of psychological factors in excessive alcohol consumption
- Have evaluated the available interventions to help people reduce their drinking

Case study

Charlotte is a 35-year-old marketing executive who works in a large advertising company. She has worked in the firm since graduating from college and has been regularly promoted. Much of her work involves networking with clients. Charlotte drank heavily as a student and, unlike many of her contemporaries, has not reduced her drinking. Drinking is part of her work culture. Charlotte often travels with her work, staying in expensive hotels and drinking late with colleagues and clients. Charlotte is proud of her ability to drink on a par with her male colleagues and to get up early after a long night and work well. Charlotte takes a lot of exercise and considers that the exercise she takes offsets the alcohol she consumes.

Charlotte and her partner are considering starting a family but have so far been unable to conceive. They have come to see you for advice about assisted conception. Charlotte's partner is clearly concerned about her drinking and thinks she should cut down. Charlotte is unconcerned and thinks she will be able to 'cut down a bit' once she is pregnant. Charlotte says she doesn't drink all that much, probably around the government guidelines unless there is a special occasion! She goes on to imply that she thinks government recommendations are rather stringent and that on the continent they are far more relaxed about drinking. You suspect that Charlotte drinks well over the weekly recommended limits and is probably a dependent drinker.

Discussion point

How would you go about assessing Charlotte's drinking behaviour and work with Charlotte to reduce her drinking?

Introduction

Alcohol is a chemical compound, ethyl alcohol, often called ethanol. Ethanol produces intoxication through its action on the brain and is a legal psychoactive drug. Intoxication leads to impairments in psychomotor control, reaction time and judgement. Intoxication also influences mood and reduces social inhibitions (Babor *et al.*, 2003).

In the UK the alcoholic content of drinks is usually stated on the container as percentage volume but it can also be measured as fluid ounces, millilitres, grams or units. One unit of liquid contains 8 grams of pure alcohol. It is generally understood that one drink contains one unit of alcohol, which can be true. However, many beers and wines are stronger, having higher percentage volumes of alcohol than those cited in Table 5.1. Furthermore, many servings are larger than the standard measures (Table 5.1).

Table 5.1 Drinks containing 1 unit of alcohol

Single (25 ml) pub measure of spirits (40% alcohol)

Small glass (125 ml) of wine (9% alcohol)

Half a pint of standard strength beer/lager/cider (3.5% alcohol)

Source: www.alcoholandyou.org

Key message

What the government considers to be safe drinking is difficult for individuals to monitor as modern drinks often contain more than one unit.

Applying this to Charlotte

If Charlotte is counting each drink as a unit and drinking large glasses of wine, or strong lagers, then she could easily be underestimating her alcohol consumption by at least half.

People can be easily categorised as smokers or non-smokers but categorising people as drinkers or non-drinkers, although just as straightforward, is not as useful. Smoking is straightforwardly bad for you, with no positive aspects whatsoever. The majority of the population in the UK and in most Western societies do not smoke. However, the picture is very different when it comes to alcohol. Ninety per cent of people in the UK drink alcohol and the relationship between alcohol and health is complicated (HM Government, 2007). Drinking a lot is bad for you but drinking moderately has some health benefits, particularly for men. Moderate drinkers have lower mortality rates than non-drinkers (Room *et al.*, 2005). Some countries ban alcohol or promote total abstinence but the policy in the UK is to promote 'sensible drinking', not total abstinence (HM Government, 2007). Sensible drinking has been defined by the government as:

> *drinking in a way which is unlikely to cause yourself or others significant risk of harm.*
> (HM Government, 2007, p. 3)

In contrast, harmful drinking is:

> *drinking at levels that lead to significant harm to physical and mental health and at levels that may be causing substantial harm to others. Examples include liver damage or cirrhosis, dependence on alcohol and substantial stress or aggression in the family.*
> (HM Government, 2007, p. 3)

Recently, the phrase 'binge drinking' has been adopted by the media. Originally the term binge was used by health professionals to describe a prolonged drinking spree lasting at least two or three days. However, the term is now more broadly applied to describe a single drinking session that leads to drunkenness (Plant and Plant, 2006; HM Government, 2007). Binge refers to the time frame of drinking. It reflects the importance of the pattern in which alcohol is consumed for health and social outcomes. It has been described by the government as:

> *drinking too much alcohol over a short period of time, e.g. over the course of an evening and it is typically drinking that leads to drunkenness. It has immediate and short-term risks to the drinker and to those around them.*
> (HM Government, 2007, p. 3)

Alcohol dependence and volitional drinking

Alcohol dependence is a recognised syndrome and the criteria for alcohol dependence are shown in Table 5.2. People learn to become dependent on alcohol. The positive outcomes from drinking – feeling euphoric, relaxed etc. – reinforce drinking behaviour. Additionally, alcohol interacts with neurotransmitter systems, which also reinforces drinking behaviour. So, psychological and physiological processes both contribute to the risk of developing a dependency. Individuals differ greatly in their neurophysiological and psychological responses to alcohol and therefore in their risk of developing a clinical dependency. Most people who drink alcohol are not dependent drinkers. Orton (2001) reported that 7.5% of men and 2.1% of women in Britain in the 1990s could be classified as having a clinical dependency on alcohol. However, dependency is not all or nothing, and many people have lesser degrees of dependency or habit.

Many people, health professionals included, believe that the only serious problems with drinking arise in dependent drinkers or binge drinkers. However, epidemiological studies have made it clear that there is a host of problems related to drinking that are not associated with

Table 5.2 ICD-10 diagnostic criteria for alcohol dependence:

Evidence of tolerance to the effects of alcohol, such that there is a need for markedly increased amounts to achieve intoxication or desired effect, or that there is a markedly diminished effect with continued use of the same amount of alcohol.

A physiological withdrawal state when alcohol use is reduce or ceased, or use of a closely related substance with the intention of relieving or avoiding withdrawal symptoms.

Persisting with alcohol use despite clear evidence of harmful consequences as evidenced by continued use when the person was actually aware of, or could be expected to have been aware of, the nature and extent of harm.

Preoccupation with alcohol use, as manifested by important alternative pleasures or interests being given up or reduced because of alcohol use; or a great deal of time being spent in activities necessary to obtain alcohol, consume it, or recover from its effects.

Impaired capacity to control drinking behaviour in terms of its onset, termination or level of use, as evidenced by alcohol being often taken in larger amounts or over a longer period than intended, or any unsuccessful effort or persistent desire to cut down or control alcohol use.

A strong desire or compulsion to use alcohol.

Source: Adapted from WHO (1992)

excessive and dependent drinking, including an increased risk of developing a range of chronic diseases (Room *et al.*, 2005; French and Zavala, 2007). Furthermore, Babor *et al.* (2003) have argued that intoxication is a major factor in many social problems such as disorderly behaviour, violence and crime. Intoxication is possible without dependence.

Discussion point

Consider the criteria for dependent drinkers in Table 5.2. Would you define Charlotte as a dependent drinker or do you consider her to have a non-clinical dependency?

In 2007 the government paper 'Safe. Sensible. Social' reported that 35% of men and 20% of women exceeded the daily benchmarks on at least one day in the previous week. Other studies have reported levels considerably higher than these (Table 5.3). Self-report is known to be inaccurate, and people are generally understood to be optimistic about lifestyle behaviours, underestimating drinking and overestimating fruit and vegetable consumption (Plant and Plant, 2006). People drink more when they are young (HM Government, 2007). Men traditionally drink more alcohol than women and, until recently, have been more likely to exceed their daily and/or weekly guidelines, even though those guidelines are higher than those recommended for women (Thirlaway and Upton, 2009). However, it appears that women are starting to drink as much as men. Table 5.3 indicates that, in 2006, women living in England were just as likely as men to exceed their daily limit, whereas in Wales in 2008 the traditional gender difference in drinking was still apparent. In Scotland there are no recent reports of daily drinking patterns, although their 2005 survey indicates that weekly drinking levels are reducing. In Ireland, weekly drinking in men reduced slightly in 2005/06 but increased slightly in women. The picture of gender-related drinking in the UK is difficult to interpret. On balance it is fair to say that women are drinking more than they used to. As this is cross-sectional data it is difficult to tell whether younger women will continue to drink as much alcohol as their male counterparts as they age.

Key message

Young to middle-aged women are drinking more than they did in previous generations, increasing their risk of developing alcohol-related conditions.

Table 5.3 Drinking prevalence rates in men and women

Source of data	% of men reporting > 4 units of alcohol on at least one day in the previous week	% of women reporting > 3 units of alcohol on at least one day in the previous week	% of men reporting binge drinking in the previous week	% of women reporting binge drinking in the previous week	% of men reporting exceeding weekly limits	% of women reporting exceeding weekly limits
Health Survey England 2006 (Craig and Mindell, 2008)	57%	57%	34%	28%	No data available	No data available
Scottish Health Survey 2003 (Scotland Executive, 2005)	No data available	No data available	No data available	No data available	18%	7%
Welsh Health Survey 2008 (Welsh Assembly Government, 2009)	52%	38%	35%	22%	No data available	No data available
Northern Ireland Health and Social Wellbeing Survey 2005/6 (Central Survey Unit, 2007)	No data available	No data available	No data available	No data available	23%	15%

A number of authors and surveys have expressed concern about the increased levels of drinking in young women (HM Government, 2007; News, 2007). Plant and Plant (2006) suggest that the high levels of binge drinking reported by young British women is unusual and has not been reported in the majority of other Western countries. A number of explanations for the high levels of binge drinking in young British women have been proposed, although there is little evidence to support any of these hypotheses. It has been suggested that women in the UK have more social freedom than women in other countries and that alcohol advertising has been especially targeted at young women (Plant and Plant, 2006). The policy document 'Safe. Sensible. Social' (HM Government, 2007) suggests that agencies should be working to make drunkenness unacceptable, but it would appear that drunkenness is becoming more socially acceptable for young women in the UK. Whatever the reasons for the surge of drinking in young women, health professionals are alarmed (News, 2007) about the potential consequences in terms of later health problems and are anxious to evaluate whether this is an acute feature of young adult life in women who will then reduce their drinking in later life or whether this trend of increased drinking in young women will persist through the life course (HM Government, 2007).

Applying this to Charlotte

Charlotte clearly thinks it is acceptable for her to drink a lot and has not yet reduced her drinking as she ages. She does acknowledge that she should reduce her drinking if she were to become pregnant. The average age of pregnancy has risen considerably, so if pregnancy does trigger a reduction in drinking in women it will be coming far later for the current generation of women.

In England in 1999, men and women from all minority groups, except the Irish, reported drinking less than the indigenous population. People from ethnic minority groups were far more likely to report that they were non-drinkers; 30% of Chinese men, 33% of Indian men and over 90% of Pakistani and Bangladeshi men were non-drinkers. The percentage of non-drinkers was even higher among women from all ethnic minorities, with 99% of Bangladeshi women being non-drinkers. Erens and Laiho (1999) reflect that social norms might result in some under-reporting of drinking, particularly among minority groups that prohibit alcohol such as Muslim communities. These data are now 10 years out of date and it is probable that the picture may be changing. When we consider the change in female drinking habits over a similar period, these figures should be viewed with considerable caution. It is possible that older people from ethnic minorities are maintaining the habits that they practised 10 years ago but younger people may well have different attitudes and practices from their parents and grandparents.

Unlike smoking, no straightforward linear socio-economic patterns in drinking emerge. We see different socio-economic effects on patterns of drinking in men and women. Whereas men at the lower end of the socio-economic scale are more likely to 'binge' drink than their professional or managerial counterparts, in women there is either no socio-economic influence on drinking reported or professional/managerial women are found to drink more.

> ## Key message
>
> Drinking is profoundly cultural because some ethnic minority groups barely drink. The most worrying cultural trend in recent years is the drinking habits of women, which appear to be undergoing a cultural revolution not apparent in men.

Government recommendations

Sensible drinking

In 2007 in the policy document 'Safe. Sensible. Social' the government recommended that:

- *Adult women should not regularly drink more than 2-3 units of alcohol a day;*
- *Adult men should not regularly drink more than 3-4 units of alcohol a day; and*
- *Pregnant women or women trying to conceive should avoid drinking alcohol. If they do choose to drink, to protect the baby they should not drink more than 1-2 units of alcohol once or twice a week.*
  (HM Government, 2007, p. 3)

The weekly guidelines of 14 units a week for women and 21 units a week for men are probably more well understood by the general public than these new daily guidelines, conceived to highlight the importance of avoiding 'binge drinking' (Anderson *et al.*, 1993).

Harmful drinking

The government defines harmful drinking for women as drinking more than six units a day or over 35 units a week. Harmful drinking for men is defined as more than eight units a day or over 50 units a week (HM Government, 2007).

Hazardous drinking

Intakes between the upper sensible limits of 14 and 21 units for women and men, respectively, and harmful drinking levels are considered hazardous (Anderson, 1993).

Binge drinking

There is much debate about what binge drinking is. Is it the number of units you consume, the alcohol content of your blood or the degree of drunkenness you experience that best defines binge drinking? Units consumed is usual in most policy documents and drinking more than double the daily safe limits in one session is usually considered a 'binge'. However, it must be acknowledged that many individuals would not consider 6-8 units in an evening to constitute binge drinking, particularly if it doesn't result in them feeling particularly drunk (Plant and Plant, 2006). On the other hand, more than six or eight units (depending on your sex) is enough to significantly increase your risk of cardiovascular events (Room *et al.*, 2005).

Trends in binge drinking are usually identified in surveys by measuring those drinking over 6 units a day for women or 8 units a day for men. In practice, many binge drinkers are drinking substantially more than this level or drink this amount rapidly, which leads to the harm linked to drunkenness.
(HM Government, 2007, p. 3)

Applying this to Charlotte

In common with many other people, Charlotte considers the government recommendations for sensible drinking to be rather stringent and probably erring on the side of caution.

Health consequences of drinking

The relationship between drinking and health is complicated. Viewed overall, the effects of alcohol on health are predominantly negative. However, alcohol can have positive effects on health outcomes when consumed moderately (Room *et al.*, 2005; French and Zavala, 2007).

Indirect health consequences of drinking

People under the influence of alcohol are more likely to be aggressive and behave violently, hurting other people and themselves (HM Government, 2007; Room *et al.*, 2005; Plant and Plant, 2006). Almost half of the incidences of domestic violence are caused by people under the influence of alcohol. HM Government (2007) report that amongst young people who binge drink a quarter become involved in anti-social or disorderly behaviour (HM Government, 2007). Drinking also has the potential to make people more vulnerable to crime. Fifteen per cent of rape victims recorded by the 2001 British Crime Survey were raped when they were under the influence of alcohol. Heavy drinking has also been linked to increased numbers of sexual partners (see Chapter 7), which increases the risk of sex-related infections.

People who are intoxicated are also more likely to have accidents. Car accidents are the most common form of unintentional alcohol-related injury (Room *et al.*, 2005). The World Health Organisation (WHO, 2002) estimate that 20% of car accidents worldwide are alcohol related. In the UK in 2005, 6% of road casualties and 17% of all road deaths occurred when someone was drink-driving (HM Government, 2007). In the UK, where drink-driving laws are relatively stringent, from 1980 to 1999 the number of people killed or seriously injured annually in drink-driving incidents fell from 9,000 to fewer than 3,000, which is a significant reduction in alcohol-related incidents. However, the number of people killed or seriously injured in drink-driving incidents over the past 10 years has stabilised and new strategies to reduce such unnecessary fatalities may be needed (HM Government, 2007).

Key message

Alcohol not only harms people physiologically, but through its intoxicating effects it puts people at risk of violent and accidental injury.

Direct consequences of drinking

Alcohol has been found to increase the risk of over 60 medical conditions (Room *et al.*, 2005). The relationship between alcohol consumption and cardiovascular health is not linear; often it is the pattern of drinking, that is important. Patterns of drinking, especially irregular, heavy drinking, have been linked to an increase risk of coronary heart disease, stroke and diabetes even when the overall volume of alcohol intake is low (Room *et al.*, 2005). Conversely, regular low to moderate alcohol consumption is associated with a reduced risk of cardiovascular disease. Another drinking pattern that appears positive for cardiovascular disease is drinking with meals (Room *et al.*, 2005). French and Zavala (2007) reported that there is a J-shaped relationship between drinking and total mortality, with moderate drinkers having the lowest mortality rates, heavy drinkers the highest and abstainers/light drinkers somewhere in between. In other diseases a linear relationship between alcohol consumption and disease does exist. Breast cancer risk increases linearly with increased alcohol consumption, with 10 grams of alcohol a day increasing the relative risk of breast cancer by 9%. A daily consumption of between 30 and 60 grams a day increases the relative risk by 41% (Cancer Research UK, 2002). Depression, epilepsy and alcohol addiction can all be caused by excessive drinking (Room *et al.*, 2005; HM Government, 2007; Plant and Plant, 2006). Furthermore, drinking can make existing psychological conditions such as depression or anxiety worse.

The disorders most people think of as being caused by alcohol are liver diseases, but many people who have liver disorders are not heavy drinkers. Only 39% of cases of liver cirrhosis are alcohol related. In 2005, 4,160 people in England and Wales died from alcoholic liver disease (HM Government, 2007). This is a 41% rise since 1999 when 2,954 people died from alcoholic liver disease.

In England and Wales, alcohol-related injury or illness accounts for 180,000 hospital admissions a year (HM Government, 2007). Alcohol-related deaths in the UK have more than doubled between 1991 and 2006, from 6.9% to 13.4% per 100,000 (ONS, 2008). A summary of the major disease and injury conditions related to alcohol and the percentage of incidents that are attributable to alcohol is presented in Table 5.4.

One area of concern is the number of people living with chronic diseases who regularly drink above the sensible drinking guidelines. Many people with diseases such as diabetes, coronary heart disease and hypertension where alcohol is implicated in the aetiology and progression of the disease continue to drink beyond their diagnosis (see Table 5.5).

Key message

Alcohol plays a part in the development and progression of a large number of serious diseases.

Measuring drinking

Population levels of drinking can be estimated from per capita consumption, which is basically an estimate of all the alcohol produced (minus all alcohol exports) and imported into a country divided by the number of adults living there. Per capita consumption is a crude measure that is useful for international comparisons and for monitoring population consumption

Table 5.4 Major disease and injury conditions related to alcohol. Diseases are listed in order, with those with the highest percentage of alcohol involvement listed first

Disease or injury
Alcohol use disorders
Cirrhosis of the liver
Oesophageal cancer
Liver cancer
Homicide
Motor vehicle accidents
Mouth and oropharynx cancers
Epilepsy
Poisonings
Self-inflicted injuries
Drownings
Haemorrhagic stroke
Breast cancer
Falls
Ischaemic heart disease
Unipolar depressive disorders
Diabetes
Ischaemic stroke

Table 5.5 Percentage of people not drinking sensibly despite diagnosis

Condition	Men	Women
Hypertension	42	10
CHD	34	6
Stroke	33	7
Diabetes	35	8
Kidney disease	26	6
Depression	42	16

Source: Safe. Sensible. Social. The Next Steps in the National Alchohol Strategy., Department of Health and The Home Office (2007), © Crown copyright 2007. Reproduced under the terms of the Click-Use Licence

over time. However, it tells us little about who is drinking within that population or anything about how they drink. Collecting data from individuals provides more useful information about drinking. Physiological measures such as a urine test provide an objective measure of alcohol levels and some indication about drunkenness, but individual differences in alcohol tolerance will influence the levels of drunkenness displayed. Surveys are probably both the most common and also the most problematic way to collect data about drinking. Surveys can tell us a lot about who is drinking and on patterns and volume of consumption, and can enable comparisons over time. They are a useful way of evaluating the effectiveness of alcohol intervention strategies. However, non-response bias is a potential problem for drinking surveys, which usually achieve response rates of about 60%. It is plausible that the types of people who do not complete surveys about drinking are different in their drinking from the types of people who do complete surveys and this introduces a serious bias. Furthermore, it is well established that people completing surveys about their drinking tend to underestimate the amount of alcohol that they consume (Plant and Plant, 2006). Nevertheless, survey estimates of alcohol consumption do predict alcohol-related conditions, which suggests that they do at least place people in an appropriate place in the drinking continuum (Room *et al.*, 2005). A summary of the strategies available to measure drinking is provided in Table 5.6.

Key message

Reliable ways of measuring drinking at one point in time are available but measuring drinking patterns is more difficult and prone to error.

It is possible to assess drinking through questionnaires, and several measures exist. One popular measure is the CAGE questionnaire and this is discussed in Chapter 8 when assessing substance misuse.

Table 5.6 Methods to measure drinking

Method	Advantages	Disadvantages
Per capita consumption	Enables international comparisons and monitoring of population drinking over time	Crude, subject to error and fails to identify who is drinking
Breathalyser tests	An objective, acute measure of alcohol levels	Needs to be immediate, gives only limited data about drunkenness
Urine tests	An objective, acute measure of alcohol levels	Needs to be immediate, gives only limited data about drunkenness
Blood samples	An objective, acute measure of alcohol levels	Needs to be immediate, gives only limited data about drunkenness
Questionnaire surveys of drinking habits	A quick and easy way of accessing data from a large sample. Can provide information about drinking patterns over time	Prone to response biases. People tend to underestimate their drinking in surveys. Response rates to drinking surveys are usually about 60%, so information cannot be said to be representative
Interviews about drinking habits	Provides in-depth data about drinking habits	Prone to response biases. Not practical for large-scale surveys
Direct Observation	Free from response biases. Unlikely to provide data about drinking patterns over time	Difficult to achieve reliable results in drinking situations. Not practical for large-scale surveys

Applying this to Charlotte

It would be possible to get an accurate measure of how much Charlotte drank at any one point by taking a blood sample whilst she was drunk. However, this is not likely to occur unless she is arrested. Asking Charlotte to self-report on her drinking is likely to be biased as she may well adapt her answers to reflect what she knows are recommended drinking levels.

Why do people drink more alcohol than is sensible?

People in the UK have always drunk alcohol, sometimes sensibly and sometime stupidly, so fundamentally nothing has changed. Overall, the majority of adults drink at least occasionally and most people drink moderately with few harmful effects. They are many reasons why people drink: because they enjoy the taste, because they like the disinhibiting effects of alcoholic drinks and because consuming them is a sociable thing to do in our culture (Plant and Plant, 2006). Young people often start to drink as part of their transition into adulthood (Paglia and Room, 1999). In the UK, drinking is a symbolic behaviour that facilitates social bonding and peer status in adolescents. Alcohol can provide young people with a seemingly adult status (Paglia and Room, 1999). Alcohol consumption at any age can be functional, providing pleasure, alleviating boredom, satisfying the desire for sensation seeking or acting as a coping or escape mechanism.

Alcohol serves an important social function. It enhances social integration and facilitates the development of relationships (Kuther and Timoshin, 2003). It is hardly surprising that people drink most at a period in their lives which is normally associated with the development of stable adult relationships (Paglia and Room, 1999). Increased levels of drinking in newly divorced people may in part be due to the breakdown of stable relationships and the desire to establish new relationships (HM Government, 2007). Social isolation is a key factor in poor health outcomes (Cacioppo and Hawkley, 2003), so the positive social function of alcohol in enabling people to develop social relationships should not be overlooked.

Applying this to Charlotte

Charlotte started to drink a lot at college, where drinking enabled her to make friends and cope with the transition from adolescence to adulthood.

Socio-economic factors

The relationship between socio-economic factors and drinking is not simple. There is some evidence that people from the most deprived walks of life are more likely to binge drink, develop alcohol dependency and to die from conditions caused by excessive drinking (HM Government, 2007). However, regular consumption at levels above the recommended limits is more likely in people from higher socio-economic groups, particularly in women (Craig and Mindell, 2008; Welsh Assembly Government, 2009). Alcohol in our culture can be considered to have no class boundaries.

Applying this to Charlotte

Charlotte is one of the new generation of professional women who drink to excess regularly, illustrating that excess drinking, unlike smoking, is not class related.

Psychological factors

Many different psychological factors have been used to explain why people drink. Initially, it was believed that educating people about the risks of excessive alcohol consumption would change their behaviour. However, similarly to other lifestyle behaviours, there is little evidence that perceptions of risk can explain much if any of the variation in drinking behaviour (Minugh et al., 1998).

Kuther and Timoshin (2003) investigated the role of social cognitive variables in predicting alcohol use. They found that self-efficacy for controlling drinking predicted self-reported drinking. Those who believed they could control their drinking drank less. Blume et al. (2003) similarly found that low self-efficacy for controlling drinking was associated with greater levels of drinking. Williams et al. (2007) found that self-efficacy was a key factor in predicting improved drinking habits in individuals identified as drinking unhealthily in the primary care setting. Similarly, Murgraff et al. (2007) found that improving self-efficacy for the ability to control their drinking resulted in a reduction in binge drinking in young women.

Applying this to Charlotte

As a woman working in a traditionally male environment Charlotte may not feel able to refuse a drink when she is out with clients and colleagues.

Social norms are consistently related to drinking behaviour. Studies that report strong relationships between social norms and drinking behaviour ask individuals how much they think their peers are drinking (descriptive norms). Kuther and Timoshin (2003) looked at both descriptive peer norms and descriptive parental norms, and found that both were associated with levels of drinking in students, although the relationship was stronger for peer norms. Similarly, in the workplace the descriptive drinking norms within that organisation and among colleagues were strongly associated with drinking behaviours both within and outside the working environment (Barrientos-Gutierrez et al., 2007). The relationship between perceptions of peer drinking norms and individual drinking has influenced interventions to reduce drinking. An individual could overestimate the acceptability of drinking among his or her peers or may underestimate the practice of health behaviours (Ramos and Perkins, 2006). Consequently, a number of interventions have attempted to challenge individual perceptions of normative drinking behaviours amongst their peers and have met with some success (Ramos and Perkins, 2006; Paglia and Room, 1999).

Drinking plays a valuable role in socialisation. Kuther and Timoshin (2003) found that students who reported higher levels of drinking were significantly more likely to report high levels of social support. High levels of social support are important for the well-being of people and protect against a range of health conditions (Cohen and Janicki-Deverts, 2009). It is important to recognise the value of drinking to young people who are embarking on the difficult job of establishing secure adult relationships.

The evidence that understanding stage of change is useful or important in changing drinking behaviours is not conclusive. Prochaska et al. (2004) have argued that the majority of students in their study were in a pre-contemplative stage for stopping abusing alcohol and claimed that their educational strategy did increase awareness and reduce episodes of binge drinking (Prochaska et al., 2004). However, their intervention was a multi-level strategy with a range of interventions and it is difficult to conclude that tailoring interventions to the stage at which individuals are at was the effective component of such a broad strategy (Box 5.1). Conversely, Williams et al. (2007) found that measures of readiness to change did not predict either future heavy episodic drinking or future overall consumption in 312 primary care patients who drank unhealthily. They found that self-efficacy for controlled drinking predicted lower consumption and less heavy episodic drinking and concluded that interventions that support self-efficacy, such as motivational interviewing, might have greater utility than stage-based interventions for promoting behavioural change in people who drink unhealthily.

In conclusion, there is some evidence that social cognitive factors can predict sensible drinking in populations. In particular, social norms, measured as descriptive social norms, are important in understanding drinking behaviour. As with other lifestyle behaviours, risk perception appears to have little or no value in predicting drinking behaviour. Similarly to other lifestyle behaviours, the role of self-efficacy in promoting drinking behavioural change looks promising.

Applying this to Charlotte

The drinking culture in Charlotte's job clearly plays a large role in her drinking choices

Box 5.1   Applying Research in Practice

The transtheoretical model of change for multi-level interventions for alcohol abuse on campus (Prochaska et al., 2004)

This paper reports on an ambitious whole-campus approach to reduce drinking. It reports that, of 1500 first and second year students, about 70% were in the pre-contemplative stage for stopping abusing alcohol. The campaign involved multiple interventions, including:

- decreasing the availability of alcohol;
- increasing the number of alcohol-free activities;
- creating a climate that discourages high-risk drinking;
- challenging inaccurate perceptions of peer-drinking norms.

Prochaska et al. (2004) found that their multi-level intervention reduced binge drinking, police complaints, and admissions for alcohol poisoning. The most dramatic effect was on student awareness of alcohol policies, with 97% of students on the campus in question, rather than 73% nationally, being aware of drinking policies.

> **Key message**
>
> A multi-level campaign to reduce drinking can be effective but working out what was effective is difficult because so many different approaches were being used simultaneously.

Interventions to reduce drinking

The Nuffield Council on Bioethics (2007) have argued that public health policies should be about enforcement and they propose an 'intervention ladder' as a useful way of conceptualising public health interventions and their impact on an individual's choice (Table 5.7).

Table 5.7 The intervention ladder

Level	Description	Drinking example
Eliminate choice	Introduce laws that entirely eliminate choice	Prohibition
Restrict choice	Introduce laws that restrict the options available to people	Remove alcohol from supermarkets
Guide through disincentives	Introduce financial or other disincentives to influence behaviour	Increase taxes of alcohol via taxation
Guide through incentives	Introduce financial or other incentives to influence people's behaviour	Fund alcohol-free events
Guide choices	Change the default policy	Recommend sensible levels of alcohol consumption
Enable choice	Help individuals to change their behaviour	Provide drinking cessation schemes

Source: Adapted from Nuffield Council on Bioethics (2007)

In terms of drinking, current government policies are firmly focused on strategies from the final two rows of the table, guiding choices and enabling choices, although certain limited strategies from higher in the table, such as taxation on alcohol and limited legal restrictions on drinking in some contexts (driving), are in place.

Plant and Plant (2006) raise concerns that the Alcohol Harm Strategy for England ignores the evidence of the ineffectiveness of alcohol risk education and the effectiveness of taxation as preventative drinking measures. The strategy highlights policies of alcohol education and voluntary agreements with the alcohol industry which have no credence with professionals in the field. The strategy ignores advice from experts such as the Academy of Medical Sciences (2004) who argue that even modest increases in alcohol taxation could substantially decrease alcohol-related mortality and under-aged drinking. The following discussion on interventions to reduce risky drinking will consider all the levels of intervention proposed by the Nuffield Council of Bioethics in turn (Table 5.7).

> ## Key message
>
> Reducing the availability of alcohol either by limiting the outlets that sell it or by increasing the price is likely to be an effective way of reducing drinking, particularly in teenagers. However, the government persists in refusing to consider such options.

Eliminate or restrict choice

There are certain groups in the UK who would support prohibition and the criminalisation of alcohol but these are a minority voice and there is no likelihood of prohibition becoming policy in the UK. However, alcohol is illegal for certain age groups in various countries. In the US, you cannot legally drink alcohol before you are 21, whereas in the UK you may drink alcohol in private from the age of 5 but may not purchase or drink alcohol in a public place until you are 18. Consequently, some interventions, particularly school-based interventions in the US, have a goal of total abstinence. The rationale for such a stance is not only to limit damaging drinking in young people in the 'here and now' but also to reduce the risk of problem drinking later, because the earlier a person starts to drink, smoke or use illegal drugs the higher the risk of later abuse (Hawkins *et al.*, 1997; Foxcroft *et al.*, 2003). In the UK, where young people are legally allowed to drink before the age of 21, there is more of a problem with binge drinking in young people. However, many countries with equally lax laws about the age of drinking do not report the same incidence of binge drinking that is reported in Britain (Plant and Plant, 2006). Nevertheless, there is evidence that increasing the minimum drinking age would reduce drinking in young people (Klepp *et al.*, 1996).

> ## Key message
>
> The US policy, in some states, of banning drinking of alcohol in people aged under 21 reduces binge drinking in young people.

Guidance through disincentives

Taxation as a public health measure is a familiar practice in smoking. It is only effective if people drink less in response to rising price. Some people have argued that it would only be worthwhile to increase taxes if people who are currently drinking hazardously or dangerously drank less in response to the rise in tax. If moderate drinkers are more affected by a price change than heavy drinkers, as Manning *et al.* (1995) have suggested, then using taxation to decrease the risk of alcohol-related disorders may not be effective. A contrasting argument is the 'alcohol prevention paradox' (Kreitman, 1986), which suggests that reduction of harm at the population level is best achieved through the reduction of per capita consumption. There are considerably more moderate drinkers in the population, so a modest reduction in drinking in this group is easier to achieve and generates more benefit than a reduction in the drinking of the smaller number of heavy drinkers. There is plenty of evidence that people drink less if the price of alcohol increases (Room, 2004) and that those of particular concern, heavy drinkers and young people, both respond to price increases by drinking less (Sutton and Godfrey, 1995). Paglia and Room (1999) suggest that adolescents are particularly responsive to the price of alcohol and that increasing the price of alcohol would be effective in reducing heavy drinking and related harm among this cohort. Plant and Plant (2006) and Room (2004) have concluded that the power of the alcoholic beverage lobby is one reason why alcohol taxation as a public health measure has not been adopted and the public health arguments are so compelling.

Discussion point

Could higher taxation on alcohol drinks reduce drinking in those most at risk of dangerous drinking?

Guidance through incentives

Funding of alcohol-free events is perhaps the least well-researched type of intervention. It has been utilised as part of whole campus, multifaceted interventions but its effectiveness is hard to evaluate as it is usually only one of a number of interventions simultaneously rolled out to change the drinking habits of a whole community (Box 5.1).

Interventions that guide or enable choice

Early interventions in drinking

Many interventions to encourage sensible drinking are aimed at adolescents and young people with the goal of preventing the establishment of unhealthy drinking habits. The rationale for a predominance of interventions for this age group includes the indisputable fact that young people are the heaviest drinkers in society (HM Government, 2007). Furthermore, there is an assumption that 'bad leads to bad', although the evidence to support this is not compelling. As Paglia and Room (1999) argue, bad beginnings do not always have bad ends, and many people who experiment with excessive drinking in their youth are not excessive drinkers in their mid-to late 20s. Nevertheless, it is indisputable that it is in adolescence that drinking begins, so encouraging sensible drinking in this cohort continues to be high on public health agendas.

Many early drinking interventions are educational in nature. In essence these are risk communication messages and the evidence from psychological research is that improving risk perceptions will have little impact on levels of drinking. Unsurprisingly then, there is little evidence that alcohol education and health promotion have any positive effect on drinking habits in the UK (Plant and Plant, 2006) or the US (Paglia and Room, 1999). These campaigns are heard and understood because knowledge in targeted populations increases (Plant and Plant, 2006; Paglia and Room 1999), so it is not that the message is failing to reach the designated audience, rather that the message has no impact on behaviour. Worryingly, there is some evidence that educational programmes to reduce drinking can have the opposite effect and increase drinking (Duryea and Okwumabua, 1988: Hopkins et al., 1988). It is possible that young people who may be attracted to unconventionality or rebelliousness could be attracted by the described risks that are intended to prevent initiation of drinking.

There are a great many school, university and community-based programmes focused on preventing the early onset of drinking and promoting sensible drinking (Foxcroft et al.,

2003). In 2003 Foxcroft *et al.*, reviewed the effectiveness of programmes designed to prevent excessive drinking in young people and, worryingly, found very little evidence that any
of these programmes were effective. What they did find was that several studies did reduce
drinking in the short term (12 weeks or less) but that drinking had returned to baseline levels
when re-assessed later. There were some promising interventions, including the Iowa
Strengthening Families (ISF) Programme and the Preparing for Drug Free Years (PDFY)
Programme (Spoth *et al.*, 2001). Both programmes aimed to develop prosocial bonds within
the family and coping skills of the adolescent. Spoth *et al.* (2001) reported that both interventions delayed the initiation of drinking and reduced current use compared to the control
group and that these differences persisted for four years past baseline. Interventions like this
are reassuring and suggest that it is possible to intervene positively in adolescent drinking.
However, great care must be taken to identify the active ingredient in successful interventions, given the very many programmes that fail to deliver positive change. It would seem
that increasing the skills of young people (an efficacy-based intervention) and improving
their social support networks are key to enabling them to resist peer pressure to take up
drinking. Foxcroft *et al.* (2003) raise a note of caution when interpreting these findings in a
British context. The different legal position and promotion of abstinence until 21 in the US
compared to the promotion of sensible drinking in the UK may mean that successful strategies in the US may not be successful in the UK. Consequently, both Foxcroft *et al.* (2003) and
Mulvihill *et al.* (2005) in their evidence briefing for the Health Development Agency conclude:

> *there is currently a lack of review-level evidence for the effectiveness of interventions in*
> *reducing alcohol misuse in young people.*

(Mulvihill *et al.* 2005, p. 36)

One study that is unusual and interesting because it reports negative findings was based
on a social norms theory but within a social marketing context (Box 5.2).

Box 5.2 Applying Research in Practice

**A social marketing intervention to reduce drinking in college students (Wechsler *et al.*,
2003)**

This study investigated the effectiveness of social norms marketing interventions to reduce
students' heavy drinking. Advertisements were used to send out messages about peer drinking:

'Most students have 5 or fewer drinks when they party.'

Wechsler *et al.* (2003) compared American colleges where social norms drinking
marketing programmes were active with those where no such programmes exist. They
reported that there was no difference in the quantity, frequency or volume of alcohol
consumption or in measures of drunkenness or heavy episodic drinking.

However, in the colleges where social norms drinking marketing existed, increases in
alcohol use and in the percentage of students drinking only 20 or more drinks a month were
reported. It would appear that the social marketing of peer drinking levels does not reduce
heavy drinking and can actually encourage students who are drinking less than the amount
indicated in the message to drink more, hardly an attractive outcome, particularly for women,
given that the amount in the message would constitute a binge-drinking session for them.

> ## Key message
>
> Social marketing about the 'normal' drinking habits of peers appears to have no impact on those drinking more but encourages those drinking less to drink more.

Wechsler *et al.* (2003) conclude that whilst social marketing strategies are an attractive solution to the problem of heavy drinking for the alcohol industry, they are at best ineffective and at worst counter-productive and tougher measures aimed at limiting access to alcohol and controlling the marketing practices of the beverage industry are more likely to be effective in reducing drinking.

It is of great concern that there are a lot of interventions that have failed to reduce drinking in young people. From those few interventions where drinking has been reduced we need to understand what was effective.

> ## Key message
>
> It is plausible that skills-based interventions can increase refusal self-efficacy. Social support is also clearly important, so helping young people to strengthen relationships may also be useful.

Interventions to change established drinking

Many interventions to challenge established drinking are aimed at addictive drinkers. Nevertheless, interventions to challenge less serious drinking exist. As predicted by psychological research, health promotion messages that inform people about the risks of drinking are as ineffective in established drinkers are they are in early drinkers (Paglia and Room, 1999; Room, 2004; Babor *et al.*, 2003; Plant and Plant, 2006). However, there is evidence that informational campaigns and, in particular, mass media campaigns and health warning labels do have a role to play in the promotion of sensible drinking. In multi-level campaigns where an informational message is supported by programmes to support sensible drinking, decreases in drinking levels have been reported (Paglia and Room, 1999).

Intervening in primary care is the most common way for behavioural interventions to reach their audience of established drinkers (Mulvihill *et al.*, 2005). In Britain, brief counselling interventions in primary care settings are the most common way that people who volitionally drink too much will receive support (Mulvihill *et al.*, 2004). It is likely that many people who are clinically dependent on alcohol and who perhaps warrant more intense intervention are also treated in this way, and so the effectiveness of these interventions for volitional drinkers may be underestimated if participants with a serious addictive disorder are included.

Brief interventions for alcohol use are well researched. They have many advantages. They are acceptable to individuals with less severe drinking problems for whom more intensive treatment would not be acceptable. They can be administered by a wide range of health professionals in many settings and are inexpensive (Moyer *et al.*, 2002). Brief interventions, although varied, have been described by Moyer *et al.* (2002) as having the six features linked in Table 5.8. Such a format for brief interventions is also recognised by Williams *et al.* (2007) who state that brief alcohol counselling interventions generally include assessment, feedback, advice and goal setting.

Table 5.8 Key features of brief interventions

1	A goal of reduced or non-problem drinking rather than abstinence
2	Delivered by a health professional as opposed to an addiction specialist
3	Directed at volitional rather than dependent drinkers
4	Addressing individuals' level of motivation to change drinking habits
5	Being self (as opposed to professionally) directed, and/or
6	Having the following ingredients: feedback of risk; encouraging responsibility for change; advice; menu of options; therapeutic empathy; enhancing self-efficacy

Level of motivation derives from the stage of change concept which acknowledges the importance of the individual's motivational state. Self-efficacy is another key social-cognitive variable which has been consistently found to predict behavioural change. Consequently, the theoretical underpinnings of such an approach are clear. Interestingly, Williams et al. (2007) found that readiness to change did not predict reduction of drinking in their cohort of people identified in primary care as drinking unhealthily, whereas levels of self-efficacy did predict a reduction in drinking. Williams et al. (2007) argue that in the busy primary care setting, formal assessment of readiness to change may not be necessary.

Brief interventions, while following this basic framework, can vary, and, in particular, the length of a brief intervention, although intuitively short, can range from one 5-minute session to brief multi-contact interventions. Many studies have found that brief interventions can reduce drinking (Moyer et al., 2002; Mulvihill et al., 2005; Poilolainen, 1999; Williams et al., 2007) However, Mulvihill et al. (2005) in their comprehensive review conclude that multi-contact brief interventions are more effective than single very brief sessions. Moyer et al. (2002) raise a note of caution that many studies report only short-term follow-up of a year or less. Given that Foxcroft et al. (2003) in their review of interventions aimed at young people found that most of the short-term effectiveness of interventions had disappeared at medium-term follow-up, the lack of long-term follow-up of brief interventions needs to be addressed. Some authors have found that brief interventions are only effective in women (Poikolainen, 1999). However, others report equal effectiveness in both men and women (Ballesteros et al., 2004; Moyer et al., 2002).

There is a significant body of work on workplace drinking norms that suggests that changing workplace drinking norms to support sensible drinking could be key in changing drinking behaviours both in work and non-work contexts (Barrientos-Gutierrez et al., 2007). The challenge will be to develop interventions that can successfully change group-based norms. Challenging descriptive social norms in interventions with young people has been utilised with some success (Paglia and Room, 1999; Prochaska et al., 2004). Similar work-based interventions may well be a useful additional strategy for established drinkers.

Applying this to Charlotte

A work-based intervention would be particularly useful for Charlotte as it is through work that most of her drinking occurs. A change in work culture would support her if and when she decides to change her drinking.

Cognitive behavioural therapy has also been found to reduce drinking in some studies (Mulvihill *et al.*, 2005). The cognitive behavioural therapy approach emphasises the ability to exercise control, and the physiological cravings for alcohol can undermine the therapeutic approach. Furthermore, the therapist and the client have to agree on the level of control they are aiming for: total abstinence or controlled drinking (Westbrook *et al.*, 2007).

Conclusion

Many people drink more alcohol than is good for them. Drinking is most prevalent in the young, where peer group drinking has been postulated to encourage and support excessive drinking. Similarly, workplace drinking cultures in adults have been found to play a significant role in supporting excessive drinking. It has been argued that reducing the availability and increasing the cost of alcohol are the best ways to reduce excess drinking, although the government has continuously resisted calls to increase the cost or limit the sale of alcohol. Interventions that attempt to build self-efficacy for reducing drinking and that challenge perceived social norms for drinking are the best way to help people change their drinking habits within a culture that is generally complicit in excess drinking.

Putting this into action

It is going to be difficult to help Charlotte until she recognises that she is drinking too much and is motivated to change. The stages of change concept would define her as at the pre-contemplation stage. Introducing her to the idea that many women of her age drink considerably less than she does might be a good way to start.

Motivational interviewing maybe a good place to start with Charlotte. On the one hand she has the social support from her partner for change, on the other the challenges of a very pro-drinking culture at work. Removing Charlotte from a working culture that supports excessive drinking would increase the chances of successfully motivating Charlotte to reduce her drinking. However, this is an unlikely scenario. If Charlotte becomes motivated to reduce her drinking then she will need to build her refusal self-efficacy so that she can continue to network with clients and colleagues without drinking to excess.

Charlotte is in the habit of drinking a lot. If she were to succeed in becoming pregnant this would be an ideal time to change this habit and develop new, healthier habits. A major life event such as becoming pregnant upsets routines and provides an opportunity to change habits.

Summary points

- Alcohol contributes to a wide range of lifestyle diseases.
- Many people in the UK drink more alcohol than is good for their health.
- Young people are the most likely to drink heavily and to binge drink.

→

- Young women are drinking more than they did in previous generations.
- Many people will have established drinking habits that are difficult to overcome without being strictly clinically dependent.
- The availability and low cost of alcohol have been implicated in the early establishment of drinking in young people.
- Perceived social norms within university and workplace environments have been found to support dangerous drinking.
- Brief interventions for alcohol use that have a goal of sensible drinking, rather than abstinence, can be delivered by non-addiction specialists and usually include assessment, feedback, advice and goal setting.
- Brief interventions for alcohol use have been found to reduce drinking in the short term, although long-term effects on drinking have not been established.
- Interventions that develop self-efficacy for reducing drinking have been found to be effective.

Useful Web links

Alcoholics anonymous 0845 769 7555 http://www.alcoholicsanonymous.org.uk/

Talk to FRANK 0800 77 66 00 www.talktofrank.com

Drink aware Trust http://www.drinkaware.co.uk/

Down your drink http://www.downyourdrink.org.uk/

NHS: Units of alcohol calculator http://units.nhs.uk/links.html

References

Academy of Medical Sciences. (2004). *Calling Time: The Nation's Drinking as a Health Issue*. London: Academy of Medical Sciences.

Anderson, P., Cremona, A., Paton, A., Turner, C. and Wallace, P. (1993). The risk of alcohol. *Addiction*, 88, 1493-1508.

Babor, T., Caetano, R., Casswell, S., Edwards, G., Giesbrecht, N., Graham, K., Grube, J., Gruenewald, P., Hill, L., Holder, H., Homel, R., Osterberg, E., Rehm, J., Room, R., Rossow, I. (2003). *Alcohol: No Ordinary Commodity*. Oxford: Oxford University Press.

Ballesteros, J., Gonzalez-Pinto, A., Querejeta, I. and Arino, J. (2004). Brief interventions for hazardous drinkers delivered in primary care are equally effective in men and women. *Addiction*, 99, 103-108.

Barrientos-Gutierrez, T. Gimeno, D. Mangione, T.W., Harrist, R.B. and Amick, B.C. (2007). Drinking social nomas and drinking behaviours: A multilevel analysis of 137 workgroups in 16 worksites. *Occupational and Environmental Medicine*, 64, 602-608.

Blume, A.W., Lostutter, B.S., Schaling, K.B. and Marlatt, G.A. (2003). Beliefs about drinking behaviour predict drinking consequences. *Journal of Psychoactive Drugs*, 35, 395-399.

Cacioppo, J.T. and Hawkley, L.C. (2003). Social isolation and health, with an emphasis on underlying mechanisms. *Perspectives in Biology and Medicine*, 46, S39-S52.

Cancer Research UK. (2002). *Alcohol, Smoking and Breast Cancer: The Definitive Answer.* www.cancerresearchuk.org

Central Survey Unit. (2007). *Northern Ireland Health and Social Well-Being Survey 2005/6.* Belfast: Central Survey Unit.

Cohen, S. and Janicki-Deverts, D. (2009). Can we improve our physical health by altering our social networks? *Perspectives on Psychological Science,* 4, 375–378.

Craig, R. and Mindell, J. (2008). *Health Survey for England 2006. Volume 1: Cardiovascular Disease and Risk Factors in Adults.* London: The Information Centre.

Duryea, E.J. and Okwumabua, J.O. (1988). Effects of a preventive alcohol education programme after 3 years. *Journal of Drug Education,* 18, 23–31.

Erens, B. and Laiho, J. (1999). Alcohol consumption. In *Health Survey for England – The Health of Minority Ethnic Groups '99.* London: The Stationery Office.

Foxcroft, D.R., Ireland, D., Lister-Sharp, D.J., Lowe, G. and Breen, R. (2003). Longer-term primary prevention for alcohol misuse in young people. *Addiction,* 98, 397–411.

French, M.T. and Zavala, S.K. (2007). The health benefits of moderate drinking revisited: Alcohol use and self-reported health status. *American Journal of Health Promotion,* 21, 484–491.

Hawkins, J.D., Graham, J.W., Maguin, E., Abbott, R., Hill, K.G. and Catalano, R.F. (1997). Exploring the effects of alcohol use initiation and psychosocial risk factors on subsequent alcohol misuse. *Journal of Studies on Alcohol,* 58, 280–290.

HM Government. (2007). *Safe. Sensible. Social. The Next Steps in the National Alcohol Strategy.* London: Department of Health and The Home Office.

Hopkins, R.H., Mauss, A.L., Kearney, K.A. and Weisheit, R.A. (1988). Comprehensive evaluation of a model alcohol education curriculum. *Journal of Studies on Alcohol,* 49, 38–50.

Klepp, K.I., Schmid, L.A. and Murray, D.M. (1996). Effects of increased minimum drinking age law on drinking and driving behaviour among adolescents. *Addiction Research,* 4, 237–244.

Kreitman, N. (1986). Alcohol consumption and the preventative paradox. *British Journal of Addiction,* 81, 353–363.

Kuther, T.L. and Timoshin, A. (2003). A comparision of social cognitive and psychosocial predictors of alcohol use by college students. *Journal of College Student Development,* 44, 143–154.

Manning, W.G., Blumberg, L. and Moulton, L.H. (1995). The demand for alcohol: The differential response to price. *Journal of Health Economics,* 14, 123–148.

Minugh, A.P., Rice, C. and Young, L. (1998). Gender, health beliefs, health behaviours and alcohol consumption. *American Journal of Alcohol Abuse,* 24, 483–497.

Moyer, A., Finney, J.W., Swearingen, E. and Vergun, P. (2002). Brief interventions for alcohol problems a meta-analytic review of controlled investigations in treatment seeking and non-treatment seeking populations. *Addiction,* 97, 279–292.

Mulvihill, C., Taylor, L., Waller, S., Naidoo, B. and Thom, B. (2005). *Prevention and Reduction of Alchol Misuse: Evidence Briefing,* 2nd edn. London: Health Development Agency.

Murgraff, V., Abraham, C. and McDermott, M. (2007) Reducing Friday alcohol consumption among moderate women drinkers: Evaluation of a brief evidence-based intervention. *Alcohol and Alcoholism,* 42, 37–41.

News. (2007). Alcohol, breast and colorectal cancer. *European Journal of Cancer,* 43, 1225.

Nuffield Council on Bioethics. (2007). *Public Health Ethical Issues*. London: Nuffield Council. www.nuffieldbioethics.org

Office of National Statistics (ONS). (2008). *News Release: Alcohol-related death rates continue to rise*. London: Office of National Statistics.

Orton, J. (2001). *Excessive Appetites,* 2nd edn. Chichester: John Wiley & Sons.

Paglia, A. and Room, R. (1999). Preventing substance use problems among youth: A literature review and recommendations. *Journal of Primary Prevention,* 20, 3-50.

Plant, M. and Plant, M. (2006). *Binge Britain*. Oxford: Oxford University Press.

Poikolainen, K. (1999). Effectiveness of brief interventions to reduce alcohol intake in primary care populations: A meta analysis. *Preventive Medicine,* 28, 503-509.

Prochaska, J.M., Prochaska, J.O., Cohen, F.C., Gomes, S.O., Laforge, R.G. and Eastwood, B.S. (2004). The Transtheoretical model of change for multi-level interventions for alcohol abuse on campus. *Journal of Alcohol and Drug Education,* 47, 34-50.

Ramos, D. and Perkins, D.F. (2006). Goodness of fit assessment of an alcohol intervention program and the underlying theories of change. *Journal of American College Health,* 55, 57-64.

Room, R. (2004). Disabling the public interest: Alcohol strategies and policies for England. *Addiction,* 99, 1083-1089.

Room, R., Babor, T. and Rehm, J. (2005). Alcohol and public health. *Lancet,* 365, 519-530.

Scottish Executive. (2005). *The Scottish Health Survey 2003*. Edinburgh: Scottish Executive.

Spoth, R.L., Redmond, C. and Shin, C. (2001). Randomised trial of brief family interventions for general populations: Adolescent substance use outcomes 4 years following baseline. *Journal of Consulting and Clinical Psychology,* 69, 627-642.

Sutton, M. and Godfrey, C. (1995). A grouped data regression approach to estimating economic and social influences on individual drinking behaviour. *Health Economics,* 4, 237-247.

Thirlaway, K.T. and Upton, D. (2009). *The Psychology of Lifestyle: Promoting Healthy Behaviour*. London: Routledge.

Welsh Assembly Government. (2009). *Welsh Health Survey 2008: Initial Headline Results*. Cardiff: Welsh Assembly Government.

Wechsler, H., Nelson, T., Lee, J.E., Seibring, M., Lewis, C. and Keeling, R.P. (2003) Perceptions and reality: A national evaluation of social norms marketing interventions to reduce college students heavy alcohol use. *Journal of Studies of Alcohol,* 64, 484-494.

Westbrook, D., Kennedy, H. and Krik, J. (2007). *An Introduction to Cognitive Behavioural Therapy*. London: Sage.

WHO. (1992). *The ICD-10 Classification of Mental and Behavioural Disorders: Clinical Descriptions and Diagnostic Guidelines*. Geneva: World Health Organisation.

WHO. (2002). *World Health Report (2002): Reducing Risks, Promoting Healthy Life*. Geneva: World Health Organisation.

Williams, E.C., Horton, N.J., Samet, J.H. and Saitz, R. (2007). Do brief measures of readiness to change predict alcohol consumption and consequences in primary care patients with unhealthy alcohol use? *Alcoholism: Clinical and Experimental Research,* 31, 428-435. www.alcoholandyou.org

Chapter 6
Quitting smoking

LEARNING OBJECTIVES

At the end of this chapter you will:

- Understand the extent and demographics of tobacco smoking in the UK currently
- Review the health and economic consequences of tobacco smoking
- Review the stages of change model and how this has been applied to smoking, and smoking cessation
- Understand the approaches to smoking cessation at an individual level
- Be able to apply a motivational interviewing technique to smoking cessation
- Consider the development of assessment, action and intervention plans for smoking
- Appreciate some of the difficulties faced when attempting to quit smoking and how to cope with them
- Understand the complexities involved in smoking cessation programmes with special groups

Case study

Joe is a 53-year-old window cleaner who is currently working in his own business but is looking forward to retiring shortly. He has worked continuously since he started work when he left school without any qualifications when he was 14 years old. He has few hobbies but loves to play with his grandchildren in the back garden. However, more recently he has found himself getting breathless frequently and thus not able to enjoy playing with them as much as he would like. He does enjoy socialising and likes a couple of pints in the evening with his friends and family at the local working men's club.

Joe has smoked cigarettes since he was a teenager and still smokes some 25–30 per day, with his first cigarette being on waking. He used to smoke more heavily but has recently cut down. Joe has developed frequent chest and breathing problems – he often has bouts of bronchitis and recently suffered four cracked ribs due to prolonged and severe coughing. In addition to his chest problems he also suffers from early peripheral vascular disease and has a mild degree of lower limb neuropathy. Joe knows that he has to stop smoking but as he has been doing it for over 40 years and he feels he cannot stop.

He sees you in the clinic and you realise that his health is severely compromised by his behaviour and he must change it or suffer ever more serious consequences. Joe reports that he only 'smokes now and again', although you think it is much more frequent than this. Joe has now noticed that his grandson, JJ, has started acting like him, plays 'smoking cigarettes' and is refusing to eat anything other than chips and bacon butties.

Discussion point

How would you go about assessing Joe's smoking behaviour and working with him to reduce (and stop) his smoking behaviour? How would you ensure that JJ does not start smoking?

Introduction

Surely everyone appreciates the health damage that cigarette smoking causes? It remains the single most avoidable cause of death and disability in the UK and the Western world (Fiore *et al.*, 2000, 2008). If current trends continue, up to one billion individuals are predicted to die from the use of tobacco in the twenty-first century (WHO, 2008). Despite the health effects of smoking being known for over 40 years, and the health impact being publicised considerably, some 12 million individuals in the UK still smoke: 25% of men and 23% of women (ASH, 2009). Although the number of people smoking has decreased considerably, this is mainly due to the established smoker giving up. The number of young people starting to smoke remains, broadly, the same (ASH, 2009).

The prevalence of smoking is not the same in different groups; about a third of those in the manual groups smoke compared to less than 20% of the professional and managerial groups. Similarly, smoking is highest in the 20-24-year age group (about 32%) and the lowest in the over-65 years (about 14%) (ONS, 2008).

Discussion point

Joe is in the lower socio-economic class, which has the highest level of smoking in the UK currently. It is likely that many of his family and peers smoke and hence the healthcare professional needs to be aware of his cultural and social baggage. Why do people in the lower socio-economic classes smoke more? Do they *choose* this behaviour?

The UK government (along with most other governments) is determined to reduce smoking across their population through both health promotion and clinical 1:1 interventions. In the UK, the Department of Health's tobacco programme is split into 'strands', each of which, it is hoped, will contribute to an overall reduction in smoking. These strands include:

1. *'Smoke-free' legislation:* From March 2006 in Scotland, April 2007 in Northern Ireland and Wales and from July 2007 in England virtually all enclosed public places and work-places in England became smoke free, including all pubs, clubs, membership clubs, cafés and restaurants.

2. *Reducing exposure to second-hand smoke:* Legislation such as that introducing smoke-free public buildings and workplaces has reduced the exposure to second-hand smoke.

3. *Tobacco media/education programmes:* A key strand of the government's tobacco control programme is the provision of an ongoing media/education campaign.

4. *Reducing availability of tobacco products:* Price increases have been a highly successful way of helping people become non-smokers: UK budget changes to tobacco duty have been directed towards increasing the real cost of cigarettes and thereby increasing eco-nomic pressures on smokers.

5. *NHS Stop Smoking Services and NRTs:* the government has set up an NHS Stop Smoking Service. Services are now available across the NHS in the UK, providing counselling and support to smokers wanting to quit, complementing the use of stop-smoking aids such as nicotine replacement therapy (NRT) and bupropion (Zyban).

6. *Reducing tobacco advertising and promotion:* the UK has a comprehensive ban, just like many other countries in Europe and beyond, on tobacco advertising and promotion.

7. *Regulating tobacco products:* This strand of the government's tobacco control programme concerns regulating the contents of tobacco products and the labelling of packaging.

Health consequences of smoking

The link between smoking and cancer has been appreciated since the seminal work of Doll and Hill (1952). This report has been followed by a succession of studies highlighting the strong link between poor health and tobacco smoking. For example, in the UK it is suggested that some 82,900 people die annually as a result of their smoking habit (ASH, 2008). Every year, tobacco smoking kills 5 million people worldwide (Perkins *et al.*, 2008) or about one person every six seconds.

Deaths caused by tobacco smoking in the UK are higher than the number of deaths caused by road traffic accidents (3,500), other accidents (8,500), poisoning and overdose (900), alcoholic liver disease (5,000), suicide (4,000) and HIV infection (250). Almost a half of all regular smokers will be killed by their habit. A man that smokes cuts short his life by 13.2 years and female smokers lose 14.5 years (ASH, 2009).

Key message

Tobacco smoking kills over 82,900 people in the UK per year. Smoking reduces life expectancy by approximately 14 years.

In terms of morbidity, smoking has been linked to a whole host of diseases and chronic conditions, including heart disease, throat cancer, stomach and bowel cancer, lung cancer, leukaemia, peripheral vascular disease, premature and low weight babies, bronchitis, emphysema, sinusitis, peptic ulcers and dental hygiene problems, and can worsen the effects of asthma and infections (see Table 6.1 and Figure 6.1 for overview).

Applying this to Joe

Joe is currently 53 and, given his current smoking pattern and the considerable ill-health he now suffers, he will be unlikely to live until he reaches his retirement at 65 years of age. Joe needs to fully appreciate the consequences of his continued smoking.

Table 6.1 Illness associated with smoking

System	Illness
Cardiovascular	Aneurysm
	Angina (20 × risk)
	Beurger's disease (severe circulatory disease)
	Coronary artery disease
	Myocardial infarction (2-3 × risk)
	Peripheral vascular disease
	Stroke (2-4 × risk)
Musculoskeletal	Back pain
	Ligament injuries
	Muscle injuries
	Neck pain
	Osteoporosis
	Osteoarthritis
	Rheumatoid arthritis
	Tendon injuries
	Low bone density
	Hip fractures
Visual	Cataracts (2 × risk)
	Posterior subcapsular cataract (3 × risk)
	Optic neuropathy (16 × risk)
	Macular degeneration (2 × risk)
	Nystagmus
	Ocular histoplasmosis
	Tobacco amblyopia
Genitourinary	Erectile dysfunction
	Impotence (2 × risk)

(continued)

Table 6.1 (*continued*)

System	Illness
	Decreased fertility in women
	Pregnancy complications (e.g. premature rupture of membranes, placenta previa or placental abruption, miscarriage, still birth, low birth weight, reduced lung function in infants)
Digestive, metabolic	Gum disease
	Duodenal ulcer
	Colon polyps
	Crohn's disease
	Diabetes
	Stomach ulcer
	Tooth loss
Respiratory	COPD
Cancers	Lung (90% associated with smoking)
	Mouth and throat (90% associated with smoking)
	Breast (60% increased risk)
	Pancreatic (2 × risk)
	Oesophageal cancer
	Stomach
	Liver
	Bladder (2-5 × risk)
	Kidney
	Cervical cancer
	Myeloid cancer
	Urinary tract cancer
Other conditions	Depression
	Psoriasis (2 × risk)
	Hearing loss
	Sudden Infant Death Syndrome (SIDS)
	Exacerbates:
	Asthma
	Chronic rhinitis
	Diabetic retinopathy
	Graves' disease
	MS
	Optic neuritis
	Coughing, sneezing, shortness of breath
	Common colds, influenza, pneumonia

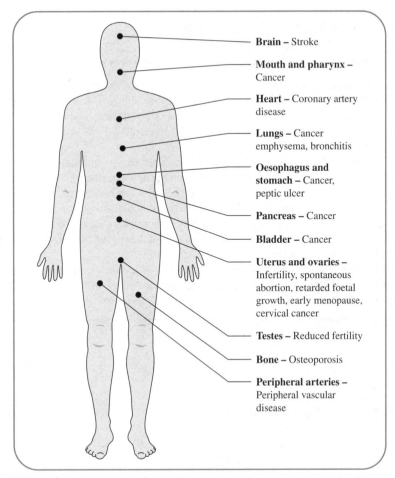

Figure 6.1 Health impact of smoking

Those who quit smoking by the age of 40 years retain almost the same life expectancy as lifelong non-smokers. Even those who quit by the age of 50 or 60 can gain several years of life expectancy compared to those who continue to smoke (Doll *et al.*, 2004). Thus, quitting smoking at any age brings with it health benefits.

Key message

Quitting smoking at any stage leads to improved life expectancy and decreased morbidity.

> ### Box 6.1   Applying Research in Practice
>
> **Smokers' unrealistic optimism about their risk (Weinstein *et al.*, 2006)**
>
> The purpose of this survey was to assess whether smokers underestimate their own risks of experiencing a tobacco-related illness relative to other smokers and non-smokers; 6,369 participants (1,245 current smokers) took part in the Health Information National Trends Telephone Survey conducted in the US in 2003. Respondents were 18 years and older, with a mean age of 47.7 years.
>
> Smokers underestimated their relative risk compared to non-smokers and believed that they had a lower risk of developing lung cancer than the average smoker. Their perceived risk of lung cancer and cancer in general barely increased with the number of cigarettes smoked per day and their estimates of their risk of cancer were slightly lower than their estimates of lung cancer. A large proportion of smokers and former smokers agreed with several myths. For example, more than half of current smokers mistakenly believed that exercise can reverse most of the effects of smoking.
>
> Taken together, the results suggest that smokers have a very imperfect understanding of the risks of smoking and of risk statistics in general. Moreover, in spite of what they may acknowledge about the risks faced by other smokers, they believe that their own risk is less.

> ### Key message
>
> Smokers underestimate their own risk of ill-health.

Assessment of smoking

Smoking behaviour can be best assessed through a subjective recording of cigarettes smoked during a defined period (usually four weeks); however, this can often be an underestimate so this has to be taken into account when making your assessment. However, if an objective measure is required then biochemical assessment of carbon monoxide levels can be assessed (using 10 ppm as a cut-off level) with specialist equipment.

> ### Key message
>
> Smokers tend to underestimate their level of smoking.

However, more important than whether a confirmed recording of smoking has taken place or whether the subjective record is accurate (which it usually isn't) is the need to assess the addiction history (see Table 6.2). Obviously, the stronger the addition the harder it is to quit

Table 6.2 Assessment of addiction to smoking

1. Do you smoke more than 15 cigarettes per day?
2. Have you smoked for more than 1 year?
3. Do you smoke low-tar cigarettes?
4. Do you smoke alone mainly, or in company?
5. Do you have a strong craving for cigarettes?
6. Do you smoke the first cigarette of the day within 30 minutes of getting up in the morning?
7. Have you tried more than twice to stop before?
8. Do you think stopping will be difficult?
9. Are you likely to encounter many situations where you are likely to be tempted to smoke?
10. Are you attempting to stop smoking alone?

Previous attempts

1. How many times in the past have you attempted to give up?
2. How long in the past have you managed to give up for?
3. What different methods have you tried?
4. Which was the most successful?

Assess whether – very addicted

– moderately addicted

– mildly addicted

Table 6.3 Assessing motivation for smoking

1. What is your reason for smoking?
2. On a scale of 1–10, how much do you enjoy smoking?

1 – hate, 10 – enjoy very much

3. On a scale of 1–10, how much do you want to stop smoking?

1 – not at all, 10 – desperately keen

4. What are the negative and positive aspects of smoking for you?
5. How would you benefit from giving up?
6. How do you feel smoking affects your health?
7. How much would you pay/give up if it meant you could stop smoking?

Assess whether – highly motivated

– moderately motivated

– not motivated

successfully. Consequently, there is the need to assess both motivation for smoking (see Table 6.3) and dependency on cigarettes (Table 6.4). These two elements should provide sufficient information for the practitioner to be able to assess adequately the individual and make their judgements on appropriate interventions (e.g. the stronger the addiction the more likely NRTs will be required).

Table 6.4 Fagerstrom Dependence Scale

1. How many cigarettes do you smoke daily?
   - 10 or fewer (0)
   - 11-20 (1)
   - 21-30 (2)
   - 30+ (3)
2. How soon after waking up do you smoke your first cigarette?
   - Less than 6 minutes (3)
   - 6-30 minutes (2)
   - 31-60 minutes (1)
   - 60+ minutes (0)

Scoring

Add up questions 1 and 2

0-1	Low dependence: stopping smoking should be easy.
2	Moderate dependence: guidance and medication to reduce withdrawal symptoms may help.
3	High dependence: guidance and medication may be required.
4-6	Very high dependence: smoking cessation will be difficult and considerable support needed. Medication to reduce withdrawal symptoms will be required.

Source: Adapted from *British Medical Journal*, 328, pp. 338-39 (West, R. 2004), with permission from BMJ Publishing Group Ltd.

Discussion point

Joe needs a cigarette when he wakes up in the morning and has been smoking for some considerable time. It is likely that he is heavily addicted. Although his motivation to quit is high, his current surroundings, along with numerous previous failed attempts, count against him. What sort of approaches should you consider with hard-core smokers? Should they differ from those less addicted?

Why do people smoke?

Before we explore how to get people to stop smoking, it is first important to see how psychologists have explained why people smoke. People smoke for a variety of reasons and a myriad of explanations have been proposed, from a psychological, social and medical perspective. The psychological explanations have been from both a behavioural and social learning perspective (see Table 6.5 for how elements from the behavioural perspective can help explain why people smoke). The information provided in Table 6.5 goes some way to help us explain why people smoke, and on this basis, how we can help them quit.

Table 6.5 Behavioural explanation of smoking development

Concept	Rules	Example
Classical conditioning	Behaviours acquired through associative learning	Having a cup of coffee and a cigarette equals relaxation
Operant conditioning	Behaviour is likely to increase if it is positively reinforced by the presence of a positive event, or negatively reinforced by the absence or removal of a negative event	Smoking is positively reinforced by social acceptance
Observational learning	Behaviours are learned by observing others	Parents or friends smoking
Cognitive factors	Other factors such as coping mechanisms or self-image may contribute	Belief that smoking looks 'cool'
Social learning perspective	Behaviour is learned by modelling and social reinforcement	Seeing parents and peers smoking – being reinforced as 'part of the gang'

Applying this to Joe

Joe tends to smoke more at the pub (although he now has to go into the pub garden to do so) and when he is around people who are smoking. The healthcare professional needs to appreciate some of the triggers that may be prompting Joe's smoking behaviour.

Interventions to reduce smoking

Evidence suggests that the majority of smokers want to stop smoking (Department of Health, 2003; Brunnhuber et al., 2007), with about a third of smokers attempting to quit each year. Just over a half of smokers do succeed in quitting smoking before they die, although for many it is too late. It can be argued that every healthcare practitioner has a moral duty to try to encourage people to quit smoking. Consequently, it is suggested that at every consultation, meeting or clinical appointment there should be professional advice on smoking, including, for smokers, how to quit smoking, in a clear and non-judgemental manner (Coleman, 2004). There are techniques, both medical and psychological, that can support people in smoking cessation attempts. It is essential that the healthcare professional is aware of the extent of these, and how they can be accessed by clients/patients.

Although it undoubtedly has considerable health benefits, quitting can be fraught with difficulties and many people report getting irritable, depressed, anxious, restless and craving tobacco. There are methods that can help overcome some of these difficulties with a range of pharmacological treatments developed to help relieve them. For example, there are sprays, chewing gum, patches and inhalers – all of which have proven benefits for the smoker (Cummings and Hyland, 2005). However, there is always a psychological element to cessation and the healthcare professional is in a prime position to maximise motivation, technique and emotional and cognitive engagement with the cessation programme.

Key message

People who quit smoking will all need some form of psychological support, whether it be from a professional or from family and friends.

Stopping people smoking

Encouraging and enhancing smoking cessation is now recognised as an important part of public health and a key role of the healthcare practitioner. Anthonisen et al. (2005) reported a 46% lower mortality rate in those who stopped smoking as a result of a cessation programme compared to those who continued to smoke. Other studies have also suggested that interventions to improve smoking results in beneficial changes in other health behaviours (Tang et al., 1997). So getting people to stop smoking can have positive consequences on health behaviours other than smoking.

Clinical smoking cessation includes (either alone or in combination) behavioural and pharmaceutical interventions and they range from brief advice and counselling to intensive support, and administration of medications that contribute to reducing or overcoming dependence in individuals and in the population as a whole (Raw et al., 2002).

Clinical interventions

The simplest individual interventions are those brief interventions that most healthcare professionals can engage in without any specific training. The Five A's model which is presented in Table 6.6 is one that is promoted for all healthcare professionals. A flow diagram is presented in Figure 6.2 which highlights the process that healthcare professionals should follow whenever they are in a position to offer guidance and advice.

Applying this to Joe

Joe has come to you and asked for support to give up smoking. You should take this opportunity to fully assess and provide considerable support and guidance. Arrange to see Joe within seven days of your first appointment.

Table 6.6 The Five A's model for facilitating smoking cessation

Five A's	Key points	Example
Ask about tobacco use	Always include questions about tobacco use	Include questions about smoking in all consultations
Advise smokers to quit	Use clear, strong, and personalised language	'Quitting tobacco is the most important thing you can do to protect your health.'
Assess smokers' willingness to quit	Ask every tobacco user if he/she is willing to quit at this time. • If willing to quit, provide resources and assistance • If unwilling to quit at this time, help motivate the patient: ○ Identify reasons to quit in a supportive manner. ○ Build patient's confidence about quitting.	'On a scale of 1–10, how ready are you to quit smoking?'
Assist the patient	• Set a quit date, ideally within 2 weeks. • Remove tobacco products from their environment. • Get support from family, friends and co-workers. • Review past quit attempts – what helped, what led to relapse? • Anticipate challenges, particularly during the critical first few weeks, including nicotine withdrawal. • Identify reasons for quitting and benefits of quitting. Give advice on successful quitting: • Total abstinence is essential – not even a single puff. • Drinking alcohol is strongly associated with relapse. • Allowing others to smoke in the household hinders successful quitting. Encourage use of medication: • Recommend use of over-the-counter nicotine patch, gum or lozenge; or give prescription for varenicline, bupropion SR nicotine inhaler or nasal spray, unless contraindicated.	Help the patient make a quit plan (see later)
Arrange follow-up	Follow-up should occur.	Arrange for follow-up within a fortnight

Source: Adapted from Okuyemi et al. (2006)

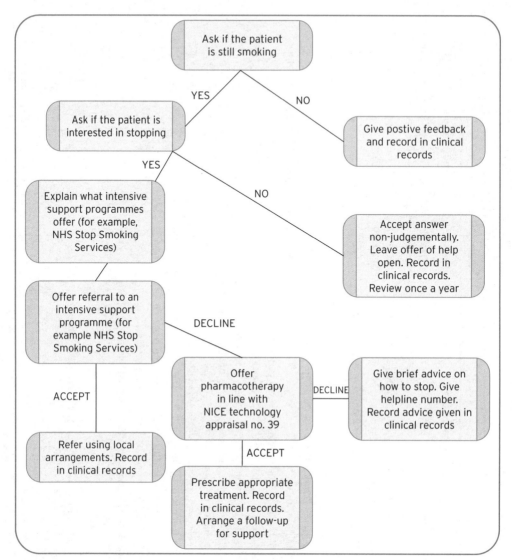

Figure 6.2 Brief intervention for smokers attending the clinic
Source: National Institute for Health and Clinical Excellence (2006) Adapted from *Brief Interventions and referral for smoking cessation in primary and other settings.* London: NICE. Available from www.nice.org.UR/PH001. Reproduced with permission.

Obviously, the 'Assist stage' can vary and these interventions are many and varied, with most (but not all) improving smoking cessation rates efficaciously (e.g. Fiore *et al.*, 2000). For example, these therapies include self-help methods, physician advice, telephone counselling, cognitive behaviour therapy, nicotine replacement therapy (NRT) and non-nicotine medication such as bupropion (Willemsen *et al.*, 2006). These interventions will be explored in more detail later.

But do patients get to know about all (or indeed, any) of these treatment options? Although a majority (some 60%) of smokers do use methods (Hyland *et al.*, 2004), not all will be efficacious and evidence-based interventions (Willemsen *et al.*, 2006). There is also evidence to suggest that many individuals, particularly those in the 'hard to reach groups' where smoking prevalence may be greater, possess limited knowledge on smoking cessation services or the treatments that are available (e.g. Bansal *et al.*, 2004). Hence, all healthcare professionals should be aware of local services and facilitate access to these services.

One attempt at overcoming these knowledge deficits was the introduction of a new health worker – the health trainer. This is an attempt at increasing the adoption of healthy lifestyles and facilitating the use of preventative services by socio-economically deprived groups. The idea is that the health trainer is recruited from the local community and works in local organisations and would hence be the 'facilitator' rather than the trainer – supporting from the side, rather than giving advice from on high:

> *In keeping with a shift in public approaches from 'advice from on high to support from next door', health trainers will be drawn from local communities, understanding the day-to-day concerns and experiences of the people they are supporting on health.*
> **Department of Health (2004), p.103**

Methods for assisting people to quit

Pharmacological treatments

Pharmacological treatments (see Table 6.7) are popular methods for assisting individuals with quitting. These include five forms of nicotine replacement therapy (gum, patch, nasal spray, inhaler, lozenge) and bupropion sustained release. A recent review (Cofta-Woerpel *et al.*, 2007) has suggested that these therapies can be considered a 'vital component' (p. 47) of smoking cessation programmes and should be available to all quitters. NRTs can, in some circumstances, double the rate of abstinence at five months plus.

Key message

There are a range of nicotine replacement therapies available and the choice should be individually tailored to the individual smoker.

Even with the pharmacological intervention, it is important to provide psychological support and encouragement for the individual smoker: the psychological factors involved in NRT use are considerable. Without continued motivation the success of NRT would be compromised. Simply focusing on NRTs may be 'doomed to failure' because nicotine is only part of the explanation for smoking behaviour. For example, behavioural techniques or de-nicotinised cigarettes may be required in order to deal with the sensory-motor activities associated with smoking.

Although NRTs are successful in assisting people to quit smoking, NRTs have not been as influential as would be predicted. Some have suggested that NRT merely encourages quit attempts by less motivated smokers who are less likely to succeed (e.g. Pierce and Gilpin, 2002). Thus, although the usage rates and quit attempts may increase, this is offset by an increase in relapse rates among those who are less committed to making a quit attempt.

Table 6.7 Pharmacological interventions for smoking cessation

Intervention	Advantage	Disadvantage	Quit rates (%)
Bupropion	Non-nicotine	Can cause insomnia, dry mouth, headache, tremors, nausea or anxiety	21-30
	Easy to use		
	Can be used with NRT		
Nicotine gum	Over the counter	No food or drink 15 minutes beforehand	7-10
• Use 4 mg if smoking 10 cigarettes or more	Flexible	Frequent use required	
• Use 2 mg if smoking fewer than 10	Quick delivery	Jaw pain, mouth soreness, dyspepsia	
• Chew each piece slowly for 30 minutes when there is an urge to smoke	Different flavours	Low compliance	
• Max 15 per day. Reduce slowly over 3 months		Under-dosing is common	
Nicotine inhaler	Flexible dosing	Frequent dosing necessary	23
• 6-12 cartridges daily for 8 weeks	Mimics hand-to-mouth action of smoking	May cause mouth and throat irritation	
• Reduce to half in next 2 weeks	Few side effects	Low compliance	
• Gradually stop over the next 2 weeks	Comes in menthol flavour	Under-dosing is common	
Nicotine lozenge	Over the counter	Frequent dosing necessary	24
• 1 or 2 tabs per hour under the tongue	Flexible dosing	No food or drink 15 minutes beforehand	
• Maximum 40 per day	Quick delivery	May cause mouth soreness or dyspepsia	
• Continue for at least 3 months and then withdraw slowly until only 1 or 2 tabs needed per day	Oral administration	Low compliance	
		Under-dosing is common	

Nicotine patch	Over the counter	Less flexible dosing	8-21
• 21 mg patch for 6 weeks	Daily application	Slow delivery of nicotine	
• 14 mg patch for 2 weeks	Overnight use	May cause skin irritation or sleep problems	
• 7 mg patch for 2 weeks		Not good at treating acute cravings	
• If smoking 10 cigarettes or fewer, start with the 14 mg patch and reduce after 6 weeks to the 7 mg patch for the last 2 weeks			
• Apply in the morning to non-hairy area of skin on trunk or upper arm			
• Replace in 24 hours			
• Use for 10 weeks maximum			
Nicotine nasal spray	Flexible dosing	Frequent dosing necessary	30
• 1 spray to each nostril as required for 8 weeks	Fastest delivery	May cause nose and eye irritation	
• Maximum 1 spray to each nostril twice per hour or 64 sprays per day	Reduces craving within minutes	Most addictive of the NRTs	
• Reduce by half over the next 2 weeks			
• Stop gradually over the last 2 weeks			
• Maximum treatment is 3 months			

Consequently, the use of NRTs has not removed the need for psychological input into smoking cessation, rather it has increased it. There are a large number of studies that highlight that some type of personal or telephone support with NRT increases quit rates, especially those using nicotine gum (Fiore *et al.*, 2000; MacLeod *et al.*, 2003). This support works by increasing motivation for quitting and remaining tobacco-free. However, most quitters attempt to stop smoking by use of NRTs alone and overlook the behavioural and psychological support required to enhance and maintain the necessary motivation (Cummings and Hyland, 2005; Zhu *et al.*, 2000). There are a number of ways of assessing motivation and these will be explored in more detail in a later section. However, three simple questions can be used:

- Do you want to stop smoking for good?
- Are you interested in making a serious attempt to stop in the near future?
- Are you interested in receiving help with your quit attempt?

These provide a qualitative indicator of motivation to stop smoking (West, 2004).

Key message

Personal psychological support is required in order to maximise the chances of success of NRT.

Applying this to Joe

Given Joe's level of smoking and the number of years that he has been smoking, some form of NRT will probably be required. You should explore the options with Joe to see which one he feels most comfortable with.

Psychological approaches

Psychological approaches to smoking cessation are important, either alone or in conjunction with pharmacological approaches, and this has been recognised since the 1960s. There are, of course, a number of psychological methods to the interventions and Table 6.8 summarises the effectiveness of particular psychosocial treatment contents (adapted from Piasecki, 2006).

Applying this to Joe

Joe may benefit from additional social support: you could arrange for him to contact a Quitline or the local Stop Smoking clinic. You may also want to discuss with his family so he obtains support from that quarter as well.

Table 6.8 Psychosocial content and abstinence rates

Psychosocial content	Estimated abstinence rate (95% CI)
No counselling (i.e. nothing)	11.2
Relaxation (muscle and imagery relaxation)	10.8 (7.8, 13.8)
Contingency contracting (e.g. 'If you give up smoking I will give you £10')	11.2 (7.8, 14.6)
Cigarette fading (reducing number of cigarettes smoked over specified time period)	11.8 (8.4, 15.3)
Intratreatment social support (support from practitioners during treatment)	14.4 (12.3, 16.5)
Extratreatment social support (support from practitioners after treatment)	16.2 (11.8, 20.6)
Other aversive smoking (negative consequence associated with smoking cigarette)	17.7 (11.2, 24.9)
Rapid smoking (i.e. smoke one cigarette, followed by another and another until sick)	19.9 (11.2, 29.0)

Source: Adapted from Piasecki (2006)

Box 6.2   Applying Research in Practice

Showing smokers with vascular disease images of their arteries to motivate cessation (Shahab *et al.*, 2007)

The purpose of this pilot study was to examine the impact of visual personalised biological feedback on intention to stop smoking.

Twenty-three smokers attending a cardiovascular outpatient clinic in London were randomly assigned to one of two groups. The intervention group received a printout of an ultrasound image of their carotid artery showing atherosclerotic plaque alongside a disease-free artery, while the control group received routine verbal feedback.

The intervention significantly increased perceptions of susceptibility to smoking-related diseases and led to an increase in people quitting smoking and intentions to stop smoking. However, the intervention only increased intention to stop smoking among people with higher levels of self-efficacy.

This study provides preliminary support for the effectiveness of personalised biomarker feedback to increase intentions to stop smoking and highlights the need to target and increase self-efficacy in smoking cessation interventions.

Key message

Personalising risk messages can improve smoking cessation.

As we can see from Table 6.8, there are a number of psychological approaches to smoking cessation. One of the earliest and most successful forms of psychological intervention is behavioural in nature. According to behaviourists, all behaviour is learnt from the environment, can be reduced to simple stimulus - response associations and, regardless of its complexity, can be described and explained without reference to internal states (motivation, emotion etc.) or mental events (i.e. perception, attention, memory, thinking and so on). Thus learning and experience are fundamental to the behaviourist approach.

Key message

According to behaviourism, all behaviour is learnt from the environment.

Behavioural approaches

Behavioural approaches to smoking cessation are many and varied, yet are usually based on the relapse prevention model of Marlatt and Gordon (1985). This model suggests that common events (whether these are cognitive, behavioural or affective) lead to high-risk situations that threaten abstinence, for example an argument with a partner or getting stressed out when driving into work. These situations can be identified with guided support by the individual smoker, although sometimes a table such as that presented in Table 6.9 may be useful to assist the smoker identify any triggers.

Table 6.9 Why do you continue to smoke?

Antecedents (before the behaviour)	Behaviour (what did you do?)	Consequences (what happened after this)
• What were you doing? • What were you thinking? • What were you feeling? • Who were you with?	• Smoke!	• What happened after this? • How did you feel?
A	**B**	**C**
Example: I was stressed out because of the children	I had a cigarette Or I went and sat down for five minutes to watch TV and relax	I felt guilty Or I felt relaxed and ready to play with the children

Consequently, it is suggested that individuals can prevent relapse by anticipating these events and learning to cope with them. This model has been taken up enthusiastically and has been demonstrated to be effective (e.g. Moore *et al.*, 2002). At its simplest, any intervention based on the behavioural perspective would explore if there were any triggers for a person smoking and then either eradicate these triggers or teach the individual how to cope with them. For example, if every time a person sat down for a cup of coffee in the morning they had a cigarette, they would be taught to have the coffee in a place where they could not smoke, or to take up some other activity during this time (e.g. reading the newspaper). Obviously it would not be sensible to substitute one unhealthy behaviour for another, so replacing a cigarette with a cream cake would not be a good idea! On the other hand, if the person reached for a cigarette every time they got stressed out with the children and they wanted a 'five-minute break with a fag' then different coping mechanisms for relaxation could be taught.

Applying this to Joe

Joe has a number of identified triggers - the pub and his friends. He needs to be taught coping mechanisms so he can deal with any potential triggers in these situations. Given Joe's smoking history - its length and its strength - rapid smoking is unlikely to be successful.

Key message

Learning to recognise triggers and cope appropriately can help in quitting smoking.

Another behavioural method much favoured in the past was aversive smoking - for example, rapid smoking and rapid puffing (Danaher, 1977). These methods involve getting the smoker to smoke intensively to the point of discomfort, nausea or vomiting. Evidence indicates that such techniques can be successful and can be used with smokers who have not succeeded with other techniques (Vidrine et al., 2006). However, there are of course associated health risks and consequently aversive smoking interventions should be used with caution (if at all).

Key message

Rapid smoking and rapid puffing are effective but can be associated with health risks.

Transtheoretical model of change (TTM)/stages of change

The most influential psychological model that has been used in smoking cessation has been the 'transtheoretical model of change' or 'stages of change' (TTM; DiClemente and Prochaska, 1982). The model suggests that change proceeds through six stages, summarised in

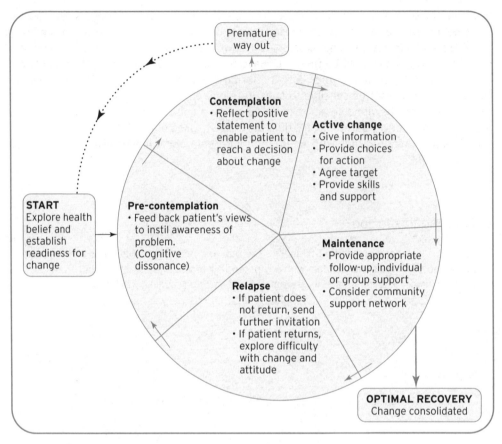

Figure 6.3 Stages of change model
Source: Adapted from Silverman and Draper (2005)

Figure 6.3. Importantly, relapse can occur at any stage, and can mean that the individual goes back to the very first stage – it is not a linear model of simple progression from one stage to another. Relapse means that you simply revert to the previous stage: you can revert to *any* previous stage.

The stages of change model has been used extensively to promote health and assist individuals in quitting smoking. This model is important because it allows professionals to identify where individuals are in their behaviour and then develop appropriate interventions (whether these be computer or media based, community or individual based, pharmacologically or psychologically based).

If, for example, an individual smokes and has no intention of giving up (i.e. in the pre-contemplation stage), the intervention to be developed will be different from that of the individual who is preparing to give up (i.e. in the contemplation stage) or has started the process (i.e. action stage). In the first case, our obligation should be to try to get quitting into the person's thought processes. We want to try to get the individual to consider giving up smoking – we want to shift them from the pre-contemplation stage to the contemplation stage. The most common method in this approach is a simple consciousness-raising exercise: increasing information about the problem and how it can affect the individual concerned. So, at this stage it would simply be a case of getting them to realise that smoking is health damaging, that it can affect them individually, and then spelling out the individual health problems. This example demonstrates that interventions have to be tailored to the individual's position in the cycle.

Key message

Interventions have to be specific to the individual's stage of change.

Interventions based on the stages of changes model usually incorporate two key elements. Firstly, it is necessary to identify accurately an individual's stage of change (or readiness to change), so that an appropriate intervention can be designed and applied. Secondly, the stage of change needs to be reassessed frequently, and the intervention modified in light of this assessment. In this way, stage-based interventions evolve and adapt in response to the individual's movement through the stages. It is suggested that such interventions are better than the 'one size fits all' model and that the intervention will be more efficient and effective than such models.

The first task that we have to do is identify at what stage the individual smoker is. This is not as difficult as it sounds and can be completed using a simple 'readiness ruler' as indicated in Figure 6.4 along with a 'confidence ruler' (see Figure 6.5) which can assist the practitioner in planning the intervention and the support that will be required.

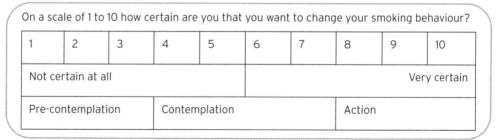

Figure 6.4 Readiness ruler for assessing stage of change of smoker

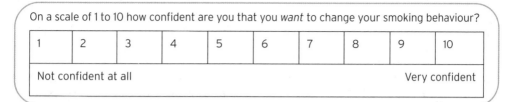

Figure 6.5 Confidence ruler for assessing individual smoker

Applying this to Joe

Joe is in the contemplation stage and you have managed to push him through into the action stage. It is important that the methods you now adopt are appropriate to this stage.

The TTM has been primarily applied to smoking (West, 2005 reported that a third of all TTM studies dealt with smoking, compared to only 13% for alcohol, cocaine, heroin, opiates and gambling) and has been *the* model for developing interventions. Indeed, surveys have suggested that the stages of change model and motivational interviewing were the main topics covered in training courses, as well as the primary theory used to explain behaviour change (West, 2005). The stages of change model has been popular with practitioners as a practical intervention guide for clinicians, and as an example of how to apply complex theories of behaviour change in an approachable and understandable form.

Motivational interviewing

The concept of the TTM can be used clinically to work with smokers. Miller and Rollnick (2002) suggested that motivation is fundamental to change and that motivational interviewing is the appropriate approach. Motivational interviewing can be defined as 'a client-centred, directive method for enhancing intrinsic motivation to change by exploring and resolving ambivalence' (Miller and Rollnick, 2002).

> ## Key message
>
> The aim of motivational interviewing is to increase an individual's motivation to change.

Motivational interviewing (MI) has as its goal the simple expectation that increasing an individual's motivation to consider change rather than showing them how to change should be the key step. If a person is not motivated to change, it is irrelevant whether or not they know how to do it. However, if a person is motivated to change, the interventions aimed at changing behaviour can begin.

Motivational interviewing is a technique based on cognitive behavioural therapy which aims to enhance an individual's motivation to change health behaviour. The whole process aims to help the patient understand their thought processes and to identify how their thought processes help produce the inappropriate behaviour and how their thought processes can be changed to develop alternative, health-promoting, behaviours. Motivational interviewing differs from counselling because it is directive – the healthcare professional elicits and selectively reinforces change talk that resolves ambivalence and moves the smoker towards change.

Motivational strategies include eight components that are designed to increase the person's level of motivation towards changing a specific behaviour. It is important to note that the motivation is specific to one behaviour, so being motivated to quit smoking does not simply transfer to being motivated to reduce alcohol consumption. The eight components are:

- giving advice (about specific behaviours to be changed);
- removing barriers (often about access to particular help);
- providing choice (making it clear that if they choose not to change, that is their right and it is their choice; the therapist is there to encourage change but not insist on change);
- decreasing desirability (of the ambivalence towards change or the status quo);
- practising empathy;

- providing feedback (from a variety of perspectives – family, friends, health professionals – in order to give the patient a full picture of their current situation);
- clarifying goals (feedback should be compared with a standard (an ideal), and clarification of the ideal can provide the pathway to the goal);
- active helping (such as expressing caring or facilitating a referral, both of which convey a real interest in helping the person to change).

Although this sounds relatively simple and straightforward and, to a certain extent, it is, there are a number of key skills that you need to employ in order to be successful in motivating smokers to quit. Some of these are presented in Table 6.10.

Table 6.10 Key skills for motivational interviewing

Skill	Comment
Express empathy	There should be no criticism or blame as acceptance facilitates change
Develop discrepancy	Change is motivated by a perceived discrepancy between present behaviour and personal goal
Roll with resistance	Avoid arguing for change or providing change – see the smoker as the source of information
Support self-efficacy	The smoker's belief in the possibility of change is an important motivator for change
Use open-ended questions	Encourage the client to do most of the talking: 'What are your concerns about smoking?'
Use reflective listening	Reflect back change talk in a statement: 'I had real cravings this morning' to 'You are a little concerned about the cravings in the morning'
Use affirmation	Use to build rapport: 'You are right to be concerned about smoking in front of the children'
Summarise	Link together and reinforce what has been discussed: 'You are concerned that your smoking may cause lung cancer'
Reframe or agree with a twist	Address resistance by reinterpreting: 'My kids nag me about giving up smoking' to 'It sounds like they really care about your health'
Emphasise personal choice	Reinforce that is the client's choice to change their behaviour
Evocative questions	
Increasing confidence	Use open questions to evoke confidence talk: 'How might you go about making this change?'
Confidence ruler	Use the ruler to ask 'What would it take to score higher?'
Strengths and successes	Review obstacles and how the client has overcome them
Reframing	'I've tried three times to quit and failed' to 'You have had three good attempts already and are learning new skills'
Prompt coping strategies	Ask for potential obstacles and putative coping strategies

Sources: Adapted from Miller and Rollnick (2002)

> ### Discussion point
>
> How would you apply some of the techniques to help Joe move from his contemplation stage into the action stage?

Developing a plan

Once the smoker is ready to quit, a plan for change has to be developed. Again, this comes from the smoker although it is a process shared with the healthcare professional. This plan involves setting goals, considering change options, arriving at a plan and eliciting commitment (see Table 6.11). It can be helpful for smokers to complete a physical plan as this will provide reinforcement and something concrete to explore when hiccups occur.

Maintaining the quit behaviour

The majority of quit attempts fail within the first week and hence it is important to follow up the individual on a frequent and regular basis – probably the first one, two and three weeks. It may also be useful to have follow-up text messages or phone calls during the first 10 days.

Following withdrawal of nicotine, there may be unpleasant symptoms of nicotine withdrawal (see Table 6.12). These physical and mental symptoms occur because of adaptation of the brain to long-term administration of nicotine. Withdrawal symptoms are normally temporary but for the first few weeks can be very distressing and may lead to relapse. It take considerable will-power and support to deal with the withdrawal symptoms and the cravings often prompt people to go straight back to the cigarettes. There is a necessity to provide appropriate psychological support during this time, and this is where NRTs can be particularly effective (see previous discussion).

Relapse

Cigarette smoking is a behaviour that is relatively difficult to change. Despite the health risks associated with smoking, relatively few smokers succeed in their quit attempts (Piasecki,

Table 6.11 Developing a change plan

Aspect of change	Comment	Questions to ask
Setting goals	The smoker's goals are the ones that matter most	What do you want to achieve?
Considering change options	Useful to provide range of optional strategies	What do you think will work for you?
Arrive at a plan	Summarise the smoker's plan	How will you go about it?
Elicit commitment	Useful to agree some immediate steps to implement the plan	What date are you going to quit?

Table 6.12 Withdrawal symptoms commonly experienced

Withdrawal symptom	Duration	Proportion of smokers affected
Light-headedness	< 2 days	10%
Night-time awakenings	< 1 week	25%
Poor concentration	< 2 weeks	60%
Cravings	> 2 weeks	70%
Irritability or aggression	< 4 weeks	50%
Restlessness	< 4 weeks	60%
Depression	< 4 weeks	60%
Increased appetite and weight gain	> 10 weeks	80%

Source: Reproduced from *British Medical Journal,* 328, pp. 277-79 (Jarvis, Martin J. 2004), with permission from BMJ Publishing Group Ltd.

2006). Even with success treatment relapse can occur quickly – with many smokers not even attaining 24 hours of continuous abstinence (Piasecki, 2006) and the majority abandoning their quit attempts within 5-10 days. In order to explore relapse, researchers have explored psychological processes such as withdrawal, urge and craving, and negative affect.

Key message

Relapse rates are high and you need to monitor your client/patient to ensure they have adequate support.

Applying this to Joe

You carefully monitor Joe over his first four weeks of quitting and then occasionally thereafter.

Factors associated with successful cessation

Although the majority of smokers want to stop smoking and some 41% of current smokers have tried to quit in the previous 12 months, the success rate is low (Taylor *et al.*, 2006). A number of studies have been undertaken exploring factors associated with successful quitting and these were often interrelated. For example, Derby *et al.* (1994) found that for women, not living with another smoker was of key importance, but for men it was increased age. Similarly, a successful quitter was reported to be an older male with higher income and smoking fewer cigarettes after previous quit attempts. Furthermore, the environment was also found to be important – being in daily contact with other smokers, for example, is associated with less success, whether this be in the workplace or at home (see Table 6.13).

As an individual's confidence grows, a number of problem situations may arise with which he or she must cope. It is in these situations that the healthcare professional may have a key role in assisting the smoker review the problem situations and suggesting potential coping strategies (see Table 6.14).

Table 6.13 Factors associated with successful smoking cessation

Positive	Negative
Smoke-free home	Multiple previous attempts
No-smoking policy at work	Switching to low-tar products
Aged 35+	
Having university education	
Being married/cohabiting	
One previous attempt at quitting	
Social support	

Table 6.14 Potential coping strategies

Situation	Potential coping strategy
When stuck in the car in a traffic jam	Chew NRT gum or have a lozenge
In the pub	Let the smokers go outside by themselves
	Stop going to the pub!
After a meal	Move on to something else – cleaning table etc. – rather than mulling over a cigarette
On waking	Use patch or gum, or clean teeth/shower immediately
When stressed	Relaxation techniques, exercise
When bored	Displacement
When anxious	Relaxation techniques
When relaxed	Displacement or avoidance
When angry	Relaxation techniques
Cravings	NRT
	Use support – either personal or professional
	Have a healthy snack (fruit, vegetables)
	Keep hands occupied
	Think positively about reasons for quitting

Applying this to Joe

You need to ensure that the positive factors associated with quitting are in place in Joe's life.

Many smokers who are willing and ready to quit struggle and often lapse at moments where some form of support would have seen them succeed. Support can make all the difference – whether this comes from the family, friends, some healthcare professional (e.g. nurse, health trainer), a support group or a helpline.

Special groups

Although the techniques and methods discussed in this chapter are of use to all populations, there are some specific groups that are worthy of further mention:

Pregnant women: Given the serious harm that smoking can do to the unborn child, it is essential that the mum-to-be gives up smoking. Pregnant smokers are often quite successful at quitting during pregnancy but it appears that those in lower socio-economic groups are least likely to quit. Success with incentives (free access to services), NRTs and particularly partner support have all been reported. In particular, it is important that the partner, if a smoker, joins the woman in attempting to quit.

Lower socio-economic status (SES) groups: There are disproportionately more smokers in deprived social groups and this is one reason for the health inequalities in social groups. Quit rates are lower in these groups and the social norm of smoking and the use of smoking as a coping strategy for a stressful environment are additional factors that have to be dealt with by the healthcare practitioner.

Hardcore smokers: These are smokers (like Joe) who have no desire or intention to quit, have made no quit attempts and have had less than a day without cigarettes in the past five years. These hardcore smokers make up an increasingly larger proportion of smokers and require considerable time and effort in order to enhance cessation. In particular, multi-level interventions aimed at both the individual and the community are required.

Adolescents: Changing behaviour among young people presents a challenge for healthcare professionals. Preventing uptake of smoking would result in the greatest population health gain. Health professionals should consider becoming involved in school-based, health-based programmes that promote acquisition of social influence skills for young people (Table 6.15).

Table 6.15 Preventing uptake of smoking by young people

Factor to be tackled	Intervention
Influence of family members (parental smoking, siblings and family attitudes)	Local, community-based initiatives running concurrently with school campaigns and media campaigns providing consistent messages
Peer influence – social influence training (community or school based); media campaigns	School influence – school-based social influence training; media campaigns
Relevance of media campaigns	Piloting or developmental work to refine messages for local populations
Changing young people's attitudes to smoking/alcohol/drugs before they experiment	Develop campaigns aimed at children aged 4-8 years

Key message

You must try to stop adolescents from starting to smoke.

Applying this to JJ

You must talk to JJ and ensure that appropriate messages about not starting to smoke are provided at school and in the family home.

Conclusion

Smoking results in significant health problems, including an abbreviated life expectancy. Consequently, it is important for all healthcare professionals to explore with their clients and patients how they can assist them in stopping smoking. In those groups at risk for starting to smoke (e.g. adolescents or those with a family history of smoking), appropriate messages about the harm caused by smoking should be provided.

In order to assist those smokers, there are a number of resources and pharmacological and psychological methods that can be used to support smoking cessation. The stages of change model and motivational interviewing are key methods that can be employed by the healthcare professional.

Putting this into action

Consider Joe's case:

- How would you assess his smoking behaviour?
- What type of smoker would you consider Joe to be?
- What stage do you think Joe is currently at?
- What do you need to do in order to move Joe into the next stage?
- Develop an action plan for Joe.
- What sort of problems do you think Joe will face whilst attempting to quit and how could you help him cope with these?
- What sort of action plan do you think you need to develop for JJ?

Summary points

- Cigarette smoking remains the single, most avoidable cause of death and disability in the UK and the Western world.
- There are differences in prevalence rates of smoking in England, Wales, Scotland and Northern Ireland.
- Although the number of people smoking has decreased considerably, this is mainly due to the established smoker giving up – the number of young people starting to smoke remains, broadly, the same.

→

- Smoking has been linked to a whole host of diseases and chronic conditions, including heart disease, cancer, peripheral vascular disease, premature and low weight babies, bronchitis, emphysema, sinusitis, peptic ulcers and dental hygiene problems, and can worsen the effects of asthma and infections.
- Despite knowledge of the health risks associated with smoking, people continue to smoke and to display unrealistic optimism regarding the impact of their smoking behaviour.
- Clinical smoking cessation includes (either alone or in combination) behavioural and pharmaceutical interventions ranging from brief advice and counselling to intensive support and administration of medications that contribute to reducing or overcoming dependence.
- Population-level interventions appear to be less effective with lower SES groups. These groups may have restricted access to individual-level interventions.
- The most influential model used in smoking cessation is the transtheoretical or stages of change model. This suggests that people move between different stages of 'readiness' for change. People can move forwards or backwards and relapse can occur at any time. However, there is limited evidence that smoking cessation programmes based on the TTM are effective.
- Motivational interviewing can be used to attempt to increase a smoker's motivation to quit.
- Lapse and relapse rates are high in smokers attempting to quit. Contact with other smokers, age, gender and previous quit attempts can all impact on the likelihood that a quit attempt will be successful.

Further resources

Coleman, T. (2004a) Cessation interventions in routine health care. *BMJ*, 328, 631-3.

Coleman, T. (2004b) Special groups of smokers. *BMJ*, 328, 575-577.

Useful Web links

British Heart Foundation 0800 169 1900 www.bhf.org.uk

NHS Stop smoking quitline 0800 169 0169 www.givingupsmoking.co.uk

Quitline 0800 002 200 www.quit.org.uk

Ash 0207 739 5902 www.ash.org.uk

References

Anthonisen, N.R., Skeans, M.A., Wise, R.A., Manfreda, J., Kanner, R.E. and Connett, J.E. (2005). The effects of a smoking cessation programme on survival in smokers with mild lung disease. *Annals of Internal Medicine*, 142, 233-239.

ASH. (2008). *Essential Information on Smoking Statistics: Illness and Death*. London: ASH.

ASH. (2009). *Essential Information: Who Smokes and How Much*. London: ASH.

Bansal, M.A., Cummings, K.M., Hyland, A. and Giovino, G.A. (2004). Stop smoking medications: Who uses them, who misuses them, and who is misinformed about them? *Nicotine and Tobacco Research*, 6(s3), S303-S310.

Brunnhuber, K., Cummings, K.M., Feit, S., Sherman, S. and Woodcock, J. (2007). *Putting Evidence into Practice: Smoking Cessation*. London: BMJ Publishing Group.

Cofta-Woerpel, L., Wright, K.L. and Wetter, D.W. (2007). Smoking cessation 3: Multicomponent interventions. *Behavioural Medicine,* 32, 135-149.

Coleman, T. (2004). Use of simple advice and behavioural support. *British Medical Journal,* 328(7436), 397-399.

Cummings, K.M. and Hyland, A. (2005). Impact of nicotine replacements therapy on smoking behaviour. *Annual Review of Public Health,* 26, 583-599.

Danaher, B.G. (1977). Rapid smoking and self control in the modification of smoking behaviour. *Journal of Consulting and Clinical Psychology,* 45(6), 1068-1074.

Derby, C.A., Laster, T.M., Vass, K., Gonzalez, S. and Carleton, R.A. (1994). Characteristics of smokers who attempt to quit and of those who recently succeeded. *American Journal of Preventative Medicine,* 10, 327-334.

Department of Health (DoH). (2003). *Health Surveys for England*. London: The Stationery Office.

Department of Health (DoH). (2004). *Choosing Health: Making Healthy Choices Easier*. London: Department of Health.

DiClemente, C.C. and Prochaska, J.O. (1982). Self-change and therapy change of smoking behaviour: A comparison of processes of change in cessation and maintenance, *Addictive Behaviours,* 7, 133-142.

Doll, R. and Hill, A.B. (1952). A study of the aetiology of carcinoma of the lung. *British Medical Journal,* ii, 1271-1286.

Doll, R., Peto, Boreham, J. and Sutherland, I. (2004). Mortality in relation to smoking: 50 years' observations on male British doctors. *British Medical Journal,* 328, 1519.

Fiore, M.C., Bailey, W.C., Cohen, S.J. *et al.* (2000). *Treating Tobacco Use and Dependence: Clinical Practice Guideline*. Rockville, MD: US Department of Health and Human Services, Public Health Service.

Fiore, M.C., Jaen, C.R., Baker, T.B. and Bailey, W.C. (2008). *Treating Tobacco Use and Dependence: Clinical Practice Guidelines, update*. Rockville, MD: US Department of Health and Human Services, Public Health Service.

Hyland, A., Li, Q., Bauer, J.E., Steger, C. and Cummings, K.M. (2004). Predicitors of cessation in a cohort of current and former smokers followed over 13 years. *Nicotine and Tobacco Research* 6(S3), S363-S369.

Jarvis, M.K. (2004). Why people smoke. *British Medical Journal,* 328, 277-279.

Macleod, Z.R., Charles, M.A., Arnaldi, V.C. and Adams, I.M. (2003). Telephone counselling as an adjunct to nicotine patches in smoking cessation: A randomised controlled trial. *Medical Journal of Australia,* 179(7), 349-352.

Marlatt, G.A. and Gorden, G. (eds) (1985). *Relapse Prevention: Maintenance Strategies in Addictive Behavior Change*. New York: Guilford Press.

Miller, W.R. and Rollnick, S. (2002). *Motivational Interviewing: Preparing People for Change,* 2nd edn. New York: Guilford Press.

Moore, L., Campbell, R., Whelan, A. *et al.* (2002). Self-help smoking cessation in pregnancy: Cluster randomised control trial. *British Medical Journal,* 325, 1383-1387.

National Institute for Health and Clinical Excellence (NICE). (2006). Brief Interventions and Referral for Smoking Cessation in Primary Care and Other Settings. London: Nice. Available at: www.nice.org.uk/PH001

Okuyemi, K.S., Nollen, N.L. and Ahluwalia, J.S. (2006). Interventions to facilitate smoking cessation. *American Family Physician*, 74, 262-271.

ONS. (2008). *General Household Survey: Smoking and drinking among Adults 2007*. Available at: http://www.statistics.gov.uk/STATBASE/Product.asp?vlnk=5756 (accessed 18 September 2009).

Perkins, K.A., Conklin, C.A. and Levine, M.D. (2008). *Cognitive-Behavioural Therapy for Smoking Cessation*. New York: Routledge.

Piasecki, T. (2006). Relapse to smoking. *Clinical Psychology Review*, 26(2), 196-215.

Pierce, J.P. and Gilpin, E.A. (2002). Impact of over-the-counter sales on effectiveness of pharmaceutical aids for smoking cessation. *Journal of the American Medical Association*, 288, 1260-1264.

Raw, M., Anderson, P., Batra, A., Dubois, G., Harrington, P., Hirsch, A. *et al.* (2002). WHO Europe evidence based recommendations on the treatment of tobacco dependence. *Tobacco Control*, 11, 44-46.

Shahab, L., Hall, S. and Marteau, T.M. (2007). Showing smokers with vascular disease images of their arteries to motivate cessation: A pilot study. *British Journal of Health Psychology*, 12, 275-283.

Silverman, J. and Draper, J. (2005). *Skills for Communicating with Patients* (2nd edn). Oxford: Radcliffe Publishing.

Tang, J.L., Muir, J., Jones, L., Lancaster, T. and Fowler, G. (1997). Health profiles of current and former smokers and lifelong abstainers. *Journal of Royal College of Physicians of London*, 31(3), 304-309.

Taylor, T., Lader, D., Bryant, A., Keysee, L., and McDuff, T.J. (2006). *Smoking-Related Behaviour and Attitudes*. London: ONS.

Vidrine, J.L., Cofta-Woerpel, L., Daza, P., Wright, K.L. and Wetter, D.W. (2006). Smoking cessation 2: behavioural treatments. *Behavioural Medicine*, 32(3), 99-109.

Weinstein, N.D., Marcus, S.E. and Moser, R.P. (2005). Smokers' unrealistic optimism about their risk. *Tobacco Control*, 14, 55-59.

West, R. (2004). ABC of smoking cessation: Assessment of dependence and motivation to stop smoking. *British Medical Journal*, 328, 338-339.

West, R. (2005). Time for a change: Putting the Transtheoretical (Stages of Change) Model to rest. *Addiction*, 100(8), 1036-1039.

WHO (2008). *WHO Report on the Global Tobacco Epidemic, 2008 – The MPOWER Package*. Available at: http://www.who.int/tobacco/mpower/tobacco_facts/en/index.html (accessed 21 September 2009).

Willemsen, M.C., Wiebing, M., van Emst, A. and Zeeman, G. (2006). Helping smokers to decide on the use of efficacious smoking cessation methods: A randomized controlled trial of a decision aid. *Addiction*, 101(3), 441-449.

Zhu, S., Melcer, T., Sun, J., Rosbrook, B. and Pierce, J.P. (2000). Smoking cessation with and without assistance: A population-based analysis. *American Journal of Preventative Medicine*, 18(4), 305-311.

Chapter 7
Safer sex

LEARNING OBJECTIVES

At the end of this chapter you will:

- Appreciate how 'sex', 'safe sex' and 'safer sex' have been defined by professionals and the lay public alike
- Understand the nature of sexually transmitted diseases and their health consequences
- Evaluate the psychological determinants of sexual behaviour and safe sex practices
- Review how psychological interventions can assist in promoting safer sex
- Consider how the (Transtheoretical Model) TTM can be used to develop interventions to promote safer sex

Case study

Gary is an 18-year-old car mechanic who is enjoying life to the full. He works hard in a local garage and earns a steady income. He has recently moved out of his parent's house to set up home with his fiancée, Debbie, in a rented flat. They have an on-off relationship but have been engaged steadily for three months now. Gary has a varied sexual history and has boasted about having more than 15 sexual partners since his introduction to sex in his early teens. Indeed, despite his determination to remain with Debbie, Gary is having occasional 'flings' with girls he meets at the local pub or night club (although he never has 'full sex' – sexual intercourse - often). Debbie is 17 years of age and has had a 'few' sexual partners (although the last time she counted, this number was over 10) but is currently monogamous with Gary. She does not want to get pregnant since she wants to complete her training as a hairdresser and is hence using the contraceptive pill. Initially when they got together Gary and Debbie did use condoms but Gary felt it reduced sensation and so Debbie was convinced to go on the pill despite her misgivings. Gary has recently experienced some pain 'down below' and has come to a GUM clinic to get it checked out. He feels that he may have contracted an STI from a recent 'fling' that went too far on a recent night out. You have recognised that Gary may be at risk from a sexually transmitted disease and have to try to promote safer sex for both Gary* and Debbie.

Discussion point

What potential difficulties do Debbie and Gary face? How is their lifestyle compromising their health? What could you do to try to reduce Gary's inappropriate behaviour?

Introduction

The first question we must ask, of course, is what is sexual behaviour? Although most people would not struggle when asked this question, further thought suggests that there are difficulties and this may have implications for assessment by the healthcare professional and any planned intervention. A simplistic, biological, definition of 'sexual behaviour' could refer to all actions and responses that make fertilisation possible. In order to effect a fertilisation, a male and female have to perform a specific series of actions and physiological responses. This may be a little restrictive, however, and sexual behaviour is more than vaginal intercourse between a male and a female. A more pragmatic definition refers to any behaviour that involves a 'sexual response' of the body. In this way the physical actions associated with sexual behaviour do not have to result in fertilisation. The definition covers all types of human sexual activity (e.g. sexual self-stimulation, heterosexual and homosexual intercourse), but it does not imply any hierarchical order among them. Moreover, it leaves each of these activities open to interpretation. In short, the above definition does not equate sex with reproduction or any other particular purpose. It merely calls attention to a certain physical response common to a variety of activities.

A final definition includes all actions and responses related to pleasure seeking. This is a modern, very wide definition which can be traced to Sigmund Freud and his psychoanalytic theory. Thus, in this view 'the sex drive' came to stand for man's pursuit of pleasure in all its forms. 'Sex' was the underlying motive of every life-enhancing activity. As we can see, when used in this fashion, the term 'sexual behaviour' becomes quite inclusive. The only question in all of these cases is one of motivation. If the behaviour is somehow motivated by the wish for pleasure, if it is prompted by an individual's inner need for self-fulfilment, if it satisfies or gives the individual comfort, if it heightens the sense of being alive – then it is clearly sexual.

Most sexual researchers use the second of these definitions. The definition does not equate sex with reproduction or any other particular purpose. It merely calls attention to a

---

* Gary is not a nice man and one intervention, many would be thinking, is for Debbie to find somebody better!

certain physical response common to a variety of activities. Obviously this definition is important for health researchers. When asking members of the population if they engage in 'sex', 'dangerous sexual behaviour' or 'safe sexual behaviour' it is important to define clearly what this covers.

Applying this to Gary

How does Gary define sex?

The majority of UK adults obtain their sexual health information from media such as television, newspapers and magazines (NSOS, 2007). This means that individuals may not be defining sexual behaviour in the way that professionals define it. Hence, when asking 'Have you engaged in sex?' or 'When was the last time you had sexual behaviour?' you may not get a consistent response. For example, a study (Richters and Song, 1999) of undergraduate student views on what activities count as 'having sex' suggested that a small proportion (7%) regarded tongue kissing as having sex, 30% regarded touching or stroking, 54% regarded oral sex without orgasm, 58% regarded oral sex with orgasm, as having sex. Over 99% thought that vaginal intercourse was sex, whereas 90% thought that anal intercourse was sex. This suggests that non-coital sex may not be defined as sex by certain key groups – younger respondents. Accordingly, the definitions of 'sex', 'sexual activity' and 'risky sexual behaviour' need to be extended and clearly defined, for both the healthcare professional and the individual.

A more recent study of undergraduates found an approximately similar pattern but approached it from a different perspective. Hence, Chambers (2007) reported that 60% of students did not regard oral sex as 'sex'. Supporting this is the finding that between 10% and 30% of virgins have engaged in oral sex as a means of maintaining virginity (Bruckner and Bearman, 2005). It is possible that individuals who engage in oral sex, but do not consider it 'sex', may not associate the acts with the potential health risks they can bring (Chambers, 2007). In fact, anecdotal evidence suggests that teenagers may engage in oral sex as a means of reducing sexually transmitted infections (STIs) and HIV risk (Barrett, 2004), despite the fact that it can bring STIs with it. Furthermore, some reports have suggested that 10% of students did not consider anal sex as 'sex' (this may be a result of some considering safe sex to be that form of sexual intercourse that does not result in pregnancy).

Discussion point

Respondents may not define non-coital sexual behaviour as sexual behaviour. Discuss the types of terms your clients use when describing 'sex'. What do they mean?

Applying this to Gary

How would you ask Gary and Debbie about their sexual relations? How do you think Gary and Debbie's definitions of sex differ – what consequences could this have?

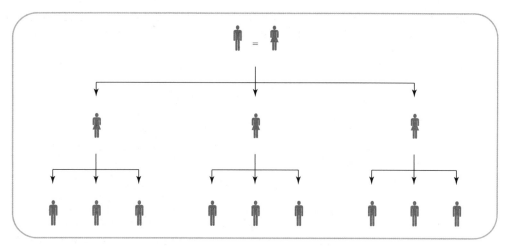

Figure 7.1 An example of a chain of sexual networking

Having sex (however this may be defined) with more than one partner in a lifetime may be a common experience. This means, of course, that calling on people to refrain from having sex does not work from a public health point of view. If we look at potential chains of sexual networking, as described in Figure 7.1, we can see that from apparently being monogamous the number of potential partners from which STIs could have been contracted expands considerably. For example, in Figure 7.1 the male has had previous sexual contact with three women, who have each had three previous male partners. So, the first male has to consider the consequences not just of having sex with an individual woman but also her partners. Hence, the female in the apparently monogamous relationship would have to deal with the consequences of 13 separate sexual couplings.

Applying this to Gary

Draw a chain of transmission of sexual networking for both Gary and Debbie.

Government recommendations

The UK government has spent millions of pounds on promoting 'safe sex' and has promoted the use of condoms as preventing sexually transmitted infections. The concept of safe sex was derived in response to the HIV/AIDS epidemic and consequently it originally focused on male homosexuals, the community where the outbreak originated, with the earliest reference to this professional term being in 1984 (Morin *et al.*, 1984). A government definition of 'safe sex' involves taking precautions during sex that can keep you from getting a sexually transmitted disease (STD), or from giving an STD to your partner. In 1985, the Coalition for Sexual Responsibility drafted safe sex guidelines to promote the distribution and use of condoms 'to eliminate the exchange of body fluids during anal intercourse or oral sex' (Lindsey, 1985).

Subsequently, health promotion officials extended the definition to heterosexual adolescents: 'judicious selection of sexual partners, the use of mechanical and chemical barriers during intercourse, and avoidance of sex practices such as those in which bodily fluids are exchanged' (Slevin and Marvin, 1987).

Applying this to Gary

Gary thinks he is practising safe sex since he is not having vaginal intercourse on his nights out. There are differing definitions of safe sex.

Recently, and mostly within Canada and the US, the use of the term *safer sex* rather than *safe sex* has gained greater use by health workers, with the realisation that risk of transmission of sexually transmitted infections in various sexual activities is a continuum rather than a simple dichotomy between risky and safe. However, in most other countries, including the UK and Australia, the term *safe sex* is still mainly used by sex educators.

Sexually transmitted infections can be prevented by condom use, but surveys indicate that individuals rarely use condoms for this preventative purpose (ONS, 2006). For example, 95% of 16-24-year-olds who use a condom do so in order to prevent pregnancy, whereas only 71% report using a condom in order to prevent infection. Furthermore, less than half (48%) of men and 37% of women report using a condom 'always'. The potential for sexually transmitted diseases arising from this lack of knowledge and appropriate usage has to be stressed. For example, the use of condoms during oral sex rather than vaginal or anal intercourse is relatively low and below 20% (Stone *et al.*, 2006) despite the fact that oral sex is a transmission route for many STIs.

The majority of adults report making no changes to their behaviour as a result of what they hear regarding sexual health (NSOS, 2007). It is clear that information and awareness campaigns are ineffective in achieving their goal and other strategies must be implemented.

There is clear evidence to suggest a reduction in STI transmission when consistent and correct use of condoms is employed. For example, a meta-analysis found that participants who reported having never used condoms had a 7.5 times greater rate of contracting HIV than those who always used a condom (Davis and Weller, 1999). Similarly, Wald *et al.* (2005) found that participants reporting more frequent use of condoms were at a lower risk for acquiring Herpes Simplex Virus-2 than participants who used condoms less frequently.

Abstinence is an absolute answer to preventing STDs. However, abstinence is not always a practical or desirable option, especially for adolescents (Berer, 2006). Next to abstinence, the least risky approach is to have a monogamous sexual relationship with someone that you know is free of any STI. Condoms can be used to avoid contact with semen, vaginal fluids or blood. Both male and female condoms dramatically reduce the chance that individuals will get or spread an STI (Collins, 1985).

However, although the 'official' and 'educational' definitions of 'sex' and 'safe sex' are well known and agreed, there is a paucity of literature on how the general public (and those at risk in particular) define 'safe sex' (Moskowitz *et al.*, 2006). A Californian study reported that most defined safe sex in terms of condom use (with 26.3% suggesting that this alone was 'safe sex'). Condom use, in conjunction with other common methods (e.g. abstinence, safe partner or monogamy), was mentioned by two-thirds of respondents. Definitions of safe sex varied across sociodemographic groups. For example, males were more likely to mention monogamy and less likely to mention abstinence. Condom use was mentioned most often by adults aged 18-24 years and tended to decrease with age. Adults aged 25-64 years were most likely to mention monogamy, and those aged 45-64 years were most likely to mention safe partner (Moskowitz *et al.*, 2006).

Key message

Healthcare professionals must recognise that people hold different definitions of safe and safer sex.

Applying this to Gary and Debbie

What would you expect their definitions of safe sex to be?

One website that provides an excellent safer sex definition is actually a Department of Health website (Condomessentialwear, 2009). The message is clear: anyone who is having sex can contract an STI: 'whether young or old, straight or gay, do it once in a while or all night every night'. The website defines safer sex as 'any sex that does not allow an infected person's blood, semen, pre-ejaculatory fluid or fluid from the vagina to get inside the other person's body'. The site goes further, to describe a number of regular and more extreme sexual practices which can place an individual at increased risk of infection before imparting advice on when it may be safe to agree to stop using condoms. This single website, accessed only after a reasonable amount of time spent searching, seems to be one of very few information sources offering a full, comprehensive definition and advice concerning safer sex. It is clear that much more could be done to encourage safer sex practices.

The National Survey of Sexual Attitudes and Lifestyles (Wellings *et al.*, 1994) examined the sexual behaviour of over 18,000 men and women across Britain and produced considerable data on factors such as age of first intercourse, sexual behaviour and contraception use. The report indicates that for men and women aged 16-24 the most popular form of contraception was condom use (see Figure 7.2). It was rather worrying, however, that many young adults in this age group reported using either no contraception at all, or potentially unreliable methods such as withdrawal or the 'safe period'. In terms of safe sex, healthcare professionals should try to encourage condom use to prevent STDs along with potentially unwanted pregnancies.

Other reports have investigated the views of both men and women. In general, men tend to report a number of negative attitudes towards condom use, including reduction in spontaneity of behaviour and reduced sexual pleasure. Surveys of young women suggest that they also hold these negative attitudes. They also tend to hold unrealistically optimistic estimates of personal risk of infection with STI or HIV (Bryan *et al.*, 1996, 1997).

Key message

Youngsters tend to underestimate their personal risk of sexually transmitted infections.

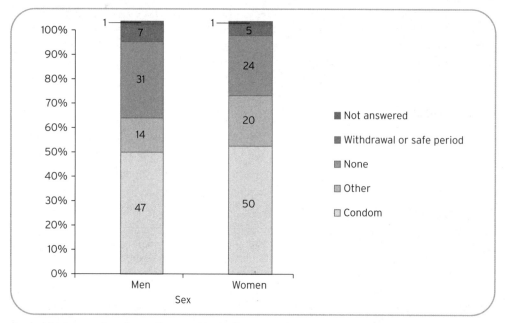

Figure 7.2 Forms of contraception used by both men and women
Source: From Wellings *et al.* (1994)

There are also a number of other negative attitudes held by women that can potentially hinder condom use, including:

● anticipated male objection to a female suggesting condom use (denial of their pleasure);
● difficulty/embarrassment in raising the issue of condom use with a male partner;
● worry that suggesting use to a potential partner implies that either they or their partner is HIV+ or has another STI;
● lack of self-efficacy or mastery in condom use.

As we will see subsequently, these negative attitudes or misconceptions have to be addressed by the healthcare practitioner in order to promote condom use.

Key message

Negative attitudes towards wearing a condom have to be confronted by all parties.

Applying this to Gary and Debbie

Gary holds a view that wearing a condom reduces his sensation. Debbie has not been able to discuss the use of condoms with Gary and has taken the simple route of 'going on the pill'.

Box 7.1   Applying Research in Practice

Predictors and confounders of unprotected sex: A UK web-based study (Fontes and Roach, 2007)

The purpose of this study was to evaluate the effects of gender, sex orientation, age, relationship status, age at first sex education, age at first sex, frequency of sex and number of sexual partners on the likelihood of unprotected sex. Participants were 10,138 men and women from the UK who completed a web-based survey in 2004.

The analysis included 9,381 sexually active respondents, of whom 58% of singles and 49.1% of those in a relationship reported having unprotected sex. Results showed that the likelihood of unprotected sex was significantly associated with a greater age of the respondent, a lower age at first sex, the absence of formal sex education and a greater number of sexual partners.

Key message

Strategies for providing sex education starting at primary school and continuing throughout secondary school need to be developed.

Consequences of unsafe sex

Sex is, for the main part, a pleasurable activity and one that has to be, for the sake of humanity, promoted. Sexual pleasure is both physical and psychological in nature and can result from a range of erotic interactions. However, it also comes with potential to do harm – sexually transmitted diseases. Unprotected sex and having multiple sexual partners can lead to unwanted pregnancies and STDs, including human immunodeficiency virus (HIV). In 2006 there were almost 40 million people worldwide living with HIV and four million new cases the same year (UNAIDS, 2006). The UK has seen the largest increases in Western Europe where annual new HIV diagnoses have doubled since 2000 (HPA, 2007a). However, STIs are not simply confined to HIV and AIDS; there are a host of other diseases that can result from unsafe sex (see Table 7.1). Young people aged over 15 accounted for 40% of new HIV infections

Table 7.1 Symptoms of sexually transmitted diseases

STI	Comment
Chlamydia trachomatis	Can be transmitted in vaginal or seminal fluids. Although chlamydia is most often asymptomatic, untreated infections can progress to pelvic inflammatory disease, and approximately 40% of women later have decreased fertility
Gonorrhoea	Transmitted via seminal and vaginal fluids and easily transmitted through sexual activity. Gonococcal urethritis causes painful

(continued)

Table 7.1 (continued)

STI	Comment
	urination and discharge, although approximately 25% of men have no symptoms. Among women, gonorrhoea can cause cervicitis, with vaginal discharge, pain with intercourse, or painful urination; however, approximately half of infected women are asymptomatic
Nongonococcal urethritis (NGU)	NGU is the most common clinical sexually transmitted syndrome among men and is characterised by painful urination with or without discharge
Syphilis	Clinical manifestations of syphilis are varied, and its natural history is complex. It can be transmitted through sexual intercourse or direct contact with syphilitic sores or rash
Herpes	Genital herpes is the most common ulcerative STI in the UK (HPA, 2007a). There is no cure, and as with other STIs transmission of herpes simplex virus (HSV) can occur with unprotected sex or direct contact with genital ulcers. There is an especially high risk of transmission when those infected have an active genital sore or an active oral cold sore
Hepatitis B virus (HBV)	Can be passed via seminal and vaginal fluids and is approximately 100 times more transmissible than HIV. About a fifth of all new HBV infections occur among men having sex with men (MSM) and people are often unaware of their status. Vaccination is the most effective strategy against HBV (HPA, 2007b)
Hepatitis C virus	The virus can be transmitted through seminal and vaginal fluids; however, the risk of sexual transmission is low. It is likely that if condoms are used consistently then sexual transmission of hepatitis C will be avoided
Human papillomavirus (HPV)	In total, 40 types of HPV can infect the genital tract. HPV-16 or -18 causes over 70% of cervical cancers worldwide, whereas HPV-6 or -11 causes over 90% of genital warts. HPV infection is extremely common. At least 50% of sexually active men and women acquire genital HPV infection at some point in their lives and may develop warts. The disease can be transmitted through unprotected sex or direct contact with genital warts
Human immunodeficiency virus (HIV)	An uninfected individual is most at risk of acquiring HIV from receptive anal or vaginal sex. Infection is initially asymptomatic. Signs of primary HIV include: fever, swollen glands, sore throat, rash on the body or face, painful muscles or joints, headache, feeling sick and vomiting, ulcers on the mouth, genitals and oesophagus. After the early symptoms, HIV may remain undetected for a number of years until the body's ability to fight infections is reduced. This leaves the body vulnerable to infections. If a person develops certain life-threatening illnesses it is known as AIDS (2007c)

in 2006 (UNAIDS, 2006). Young people under 16 have also seen the largest increase in chlamydia; the largest prevalence rates are in those aged between 16 and 24 (ONS, 2006). Chlamydia and gonorrhoea are the two most common STIs and both are the key cause of preventable infertility amongst women, and along with other STIs make the acquisition and transmission of HIV between three and five times more likely (Barry and Klausner, 2006).

In the UK, the number of reported cases of STIs has risen considerably, particularly amongst young people (see Table 7.2). For instance, between 1995 and 2003, diagnoses of new episodes of gonorrhoea and chlamydia increased by 197% and 409% respectively among men aged 16-19 years (HPA, 2008). From Table 7.3 (adapted from HPA, 2008) the increases are truly massive – a 1800% increase in syphilis, for example. Given the increase in STIs and unwanted pregnancies in adolescence, it is hard to disagree with the contention that the sexual health of England and Wales is in crisis and the worst in Europe (Evans and Tripp, 2006). Obviously, from this perspective, sexual behaviour moves from the pleasurable to the irresponsible and dangerous. However, not surprisingly, most people who engage in sexual activity are thinking of pleasure rather than any concerns over sexually transmitted diseases

Table 7.2 Rates per 100,000 of population of STI diagnoses by country (2006)

	Gonorrhoea	Syphilis	Chlamydia	Genital warts	Genital herpes
England	35	5.0	197	141	38
Wales	16	1.1	126	125	22
Northern Ireland	11	1.7	115	125	22
Scotland	17	3.7	170	135	27
UK	32	4.6	189	139	36

Table 7.3 STI diagnoses at GUM (genitourinary medicine) clinics in the UK: 1998-2007

Year	Syphilis	Gonorrhoea	Chlamydia	Herpes	Genital warts	All new diagnoses
1998	139	13,212	48,726	17,248	70,291	244,282
1999	223	16,470	56,991	17,509	71,748	261,406
2000	342	21,800	68,332	17,823	71,317	284,035
2001	753	23,705	76,515	18,944	73,458	303,169
2002	1,257	25,591	87,588	19,438	74,969	324,170
2003	1,652	24,973	96,159	19,233	76,599	346,168
2004	2,283	22,326	104,739	19,073	80,059	363,289
2005	2,721	19,248	109,418	19,830	81,201	368,258
2006	2,684	18,898	113,783	21,797	83,624	375,843
2007	2,680	18,710	121,986	26,062	89,838	397,990
% change (1998-2007)	**1,828%**	**42%**	**150%**	**51%**	**28%**	**63%**

Source: Adapted from HPA (2008)

(Philpott *et al.*, 2006). Thus, the healthcare professional has to deal with a tricky dilemma – the promotion of safe sex without denying the pursuit of pleasure. Indeed, some have argued that denying the possibility of pleasure in sexual relations, especially for women, has a negative impact on their active negotiation of safer sex (Holland *et al.*, 1992).

Key message

When attempting to promote safe sex, the pleasure achieved from sex must be acknowledged.

Applying this to Gary

What positives consequences does Gary get from his sexual relationships, both with Debbie and with his 'conquests' at the local night spots?

Applying this to Gary and Debbie

What sexually transmitted diseases are Gary and Debbie exposing themselves to?

Why do people have safe/unsafe sex?

To combat the spread of STDs the government's message is to use a condom. Research evidence has supported the contention that consistent condom use is associated with reduced risk of STDs (e.g. Gallo *et al.*, 2007) and use of condoms during each risky sexual encounter is the only efficient way to prevent the spread of most STDs (Carey *et al.*, 1992). However, in one US study some 78% of respondents declared that they did not always use a condom during sexual intercourse (Choi and Catania, 1996). In a European study, among the respondents who had more than one partner in the year preceding the study, only 52% of the men and 41% of the women declared having used a condom at least once (Guiguet *et al.*, 1994). Not only does the condom have to be used, but it has to be used effectively (i.e. properly). Hatherall *et al.* (2007) report that a sizeable minority (between 12% and 40%) applied a condom imperfectly. Given that imperfect use of condoms fails to maximise their effectiveness as a method of STI prevention, it is obviously important to address this through appropriate public health messages.

So, why do couples not use a condom? And if they do, why don't they use it correctly? Why is it that, despite the risks, individuals still take the risk and have unsafe sex? There are, of course, a number of possible reasons why this might be, and many of these are psychological in nature.

There may be some external factors to consider as well. For example, young people's sexual encounters are often unplanned, sporadic and sometimes the result of social pressure, coercion or alcohol (Lear, 1995). Early sexual activity is associated with alcohol and drug use, intimate partner violence, pregnancy and inconsistent condom use, as well as multiple sex partners (Hahm *et al.*, 2006). It is possible that the two decisions (young age of first sex and non-use of condom) are related and it may be that younger teens are less able to negotiate condom use or that younger age at first sex is a marker for other underlying risk-taking propensities. However, it is clear that drugs and alcohol play a significant role in sexual behaviour for adolescents. For example, in one study (Bartlett *et al.*, 2007) the sample reported that alcohol and drugs played a significant role in decision-making about sex and nearly a third reported that alcohol and drugs had contributed to them doing 'more' sexually than they would when sober.

Key message

Drugs and alcohol can play a significant part in sexual behaviour in adolescents.

Buhi and Goodson (2007) reviewed the predictors of risky sexual behaviour in adolescents and classified these factors under common themes (see Table 7.4).

Table 7.4 Summary of predictors of sexual behaviour

Theme	Element
Intention to have sex	• Initiation of sexual behaviour (+);
Environmental constraints	• Greater parental involvement (+/0);
	• High quality of relationship with parents (+/0);
	• Fewer rules/boundaries (−/0);
	• Increased parental support (+/0/−);
	• Greater parental monitoring/supervision (+/0);
	• Increased peer support (0);
	• Increased time home alone (without a parent) (−);
Norms	• Perceptions of peer sex behaviours (believing most peers have had sex) (−/0);
	• Perception of peer disapproval of sex or negative attitudes towards sex (+/0);
	• Perceived parental disapproval of engaging in sexual intercourse (+);
	• Self-efficacy (+/0);
	• Pro abstinence self-standards (+);
	• Negative emotions regarding sex/positive emotions towards sexual abstinence (+/0);
	• Positive attitudes toward abstinence/fewer sexually permissive attitudes (+/0);

Note: (−) indicates that this element is a risk factor, (+) indicates a protective factor, (0) indicates a non-statistically significant finding.

Source: Buhi and Goodson (2007)

A different approach was adopted by Marston and King (2006) who reported a systematic review of qualitative studies exploring young people's sexual behaviour and revealed seven themes. Firstly, young people assess the risk by deciding whether the partner is 'clean' or 'unclean' on the basis of how well they know their partner, their partner's appearance or other such 'indicators'. Secondly, sexual partners have an important influence in general. Individuals might see sex as a way of strengthening a relationship whilst, conversely, fear of physical violence can split up a relationship. The third theme identified was that condoms could be stigmatising and associated with lack of trust; they were perceived as undesirable, suggesting that their partner might be 'unclean' and demonstrating a lack of trust. Next, gender stereotypes were seen as important: men are expected to be highly heterosexually active, and women chaste. Fifth, the social rewards (i.e. penalties and rewards) influence behaviour. Complying with gender expectations can raise social status: for men by having many partners and for women by chastity to secure a stable relationship. The sixth theme was that reputation and social displays of sexual activity or inactivity are important. Finally, these social expectations hamper communication.

Applying this to Gary

What factors contribute to Gary not practising safe sex?

There are a number of psychological variables that may be important when discussing sexual behaviour. Potentially one of the most important of these is self-efficacy. Studies (e.g. Buhi and Goodson, 2007) have indicated a protective effect of self-efficacy. For example, greater self-efficacy resulted in the ability to resist peer pressure to have sex (Dilorio et al., 2001), delay initiation of sexual intercourse (Santelli et al., 2004), avoid sexual activity or risky sexual behaviour and to remain abstinent (Collazo, 2004).

Key message

Self-efficacy is an important variable in promoting appropriate sexual behaviour.

Another psychological variable implicated in the Godin et al. (2005) study was moral norm. This variable represents a measure of personal feelings of moral obligation or responsibility for adopting a given behaviour. This is perceived as a variable of growing importance in the health-related domain and has implications for the development of appropriate interventions and media campaigns.

Other reasons why unprotected sex may occur is that there may be other goals besides health. For example, sharing intimacy, experiencing belongingness and increasing one's own self-esteem are some of the goals which may override thoughts of health in an immediate situation (e.g. Gebhardt et al., 2006; Logan et al., 2003). These psychological functions served by sexual behaviour may impact on safe sex behaviour. For example, Browning et al. (2000) found, in a sample of students, that pursuit of pleasure within a sexual relationship was negatively related to condom use.

> ### Key message
>
> There are many reasons why people enter sexual relationships, not simply sexual pleasure.

Finally, psychological research on the determinants of unsafe sexual practice has usually employed the social cognition models outlined in Chapter 3, including theories such as the Health Belief Model (Rosenstock, 1990), the Protection Motivation Theory (Rogers, 1975), the Theory of Reasoned Action (Fishbein and Ajzen, 1975) and the Theory of Planned Behaviour (Ajzen, 1985). Within this type of conceptualisation, it is assumed that individuals are motivated to use a condom if the benefits of doing so outweigh the costs, and that they are able to perform the behaviour.

All of these factors have to be used by the healthcare professional when attempting to devise intervention strategies.

> ### Applying this to Gary
>
> What factors will have to be included in any intervention designed to assist Gary and Debbie?

Interventions to promote safer sex

Within the UK, the Department of Health suggested that there were a number of actions that needed to be put in place. The first of these was to develop a national campaign aimed at younger men and women to ensure that they understand the real risk of unprotected sex and persuade them of the benefits of using condoms to avoid the risk of STIs or unplanned pregnancies (see, for example, http://www.condomessentialwear.co.uk/). Furthermore, there was a longer-term strategy to ensure that children and young people were on the right path towards improving their sexual health by reducing teenage pregnancy and consumption of alcohol and illicit drugs. Developments of new resources for the health service (e.g. FIT magazine, confidential email service, websites such as www.ruthinking.co.uk or www.teenagehealthfreak.org) are all part of this approach.

Such interventional programmes aimed at promoting condom use have used a range of strategies and media, including, amongst others, lectures, leaflets, interactive games and websites, films, role-modelling, and posters. Public health campaigns have employed poster campaigns, TV, newspaper and cinema advertising, interactive computer and web programs and health promotion leaflets (see websites above; Dunn et al., 1998; Sanderson, 2000).

The theoretically derived interventions have concentrated on the social cognition models approach to safer sexual behaviour. These models have suggested that knowledge about STDs and beliefs about infection, risk and symptom severity are weaker predictors of condom use than action-specific cognitions, such as attitudes towards condom use, perceived self-efficacy in relation to condom use, the social acceptability of condom use and condom use intentions. Sheeran et al., (1999) reported a comprehensive meta-analysis of 121 empirical research studies into cognitive and behavioural correlates of heterosexual condom use. The study identified key measures associated with modest correlations with condom use:

- Attitudes towards condoms: the more positive the attitude (based on many factors, not least an individual's view on the pros and cons of condom use), the more it will result in increased condom usage;
- Descriptive norms in relation to condom use: the perceptions that others approve of and use condoms;
- Pregnancy motivation: the belief that condoms should be used for contraceptive purposes as well as STI protection;
- Intentions to use condoms: a belief based on education, practice and attitude;
- Carrying condoms: having them available for use;
- Ensuring condoms were available: not just carrying them but having them accessible;
- Communication with sexual partners about condoms: being able to discuss safer sex and condom use with the sexual partner.

Sheeran et al. (1999) conclude that these results 'provide empirical support for conceptualising condom use in terms of . . . an extended Theory of Reasoned Action' (p. 126) and suggest that these correlates specify potentially useful targets for safer sex promotion. On the basis of this meta-analysis, Abraham et al. (2002) investigated whether this had been taken into account when developing health education practice. They reported that leaflets focused mainly on the provision of information, highlighting risk, encouraging professional contact and confirming efficacy of condom use and not those suggested by Sheeran et al. (1999). It appears as if there was an evidence-based deficit: the practice was not based on theoretically conceived research. Consequently, it is important to note that the specifically tailored interventions for individuals have to attempt to overcome this deficit and develop appropriate materials.

Key message

Use psychological knowledge to improve your practice!

Only a few instances of interventions have been found in research studies that highlight abstaining from or delaying sexual intercourse (e.g. Schaalma et al., 2004; Thomas, 2000). This is surprising given that there is a growth of such a movement within the US (e.g. The Silver Ring Thing: http://www.silverringthing.com/) and smaller movements within the UK. It may be that health educators fear that their audience will be unwilling to contemplate delaying sexual intercourse. The other problem with this approach, as discussed above, is: what is abstinence? Does it mean only 'not having sexual intercourse'? Or does it mean not kissing or touching as well? Furthermore, all adolescents experience some form of sexual desire. As Berer (2006) suggests, 'The prescription of abstinence is a potential death sentence for anyone who wants to have sex if the means to make it safe, at whatever age, are withheld' (p. 7).

Shrier et al. (2001) explored whether an individual intervention based on various psychological models, including the Stages of Change (SoC) (Prochaska and DiClemente, 2002), and implemented through motivational interviewing (Miller and Rollnick, 1982) could improve condom use. The intervention they suggested began with a seven-minute video in which popular entertainers and sports figures discussed and dramatised condom names, buying condoms, and negotiating condom use, and two female adolescents demonstrated condom use to their peers. Condom use was portrayed as normative behaviour.

Key message

Portraying condom use as a normative behaviour can increase awareness and usage.

In addition to this, a series of female health educators were employed and trained in various theories and were taught to use a standardised intervention manual that outlined key points to cover, activities to perform and the motivation strategies to employ. At the outset, participants were asked about how much they needed and wanted to change their sexual risk behaviour (on a so-called 'wheel of change'). The intervention ensured that the same information was provided to all participants but the educator tried to individualise the session based on the stage of change. On the basis of this intervention, there was an improvement in condom use in that more of the participants used condoms during sex than previously. However, this is one specific example and there are many others which are based on the stages of change model.

Discussion point

Think about Gary and Debbie. How could the healthcare professional work with Debbie to improve Gary's sexual behaviour?

There are other psychological models that can contribute to the promotion of safer sex and can be incorporated into any intervention based on the SoC model. One example would be from the Theory of Planned Behaviour (Fishbein and Ajzen, 1975), which suggests that subjective norms, including peer norms, are important factors related to stage of change. For example, adolescents who perceive a greater support for safer sex are more likely to improve and maintain their own sexual behaviour (e.g. Sieving et al., 2006).

The stages of change model has been described extensively elsewhere in this book, for example how it can be applied to smoking cessation in Chapter 6. However, it serves as a useful model for developing and implementing intervention strategies for a range of lifestyle behaviours and safe sex is one of them. The stages of change model (Prochaska and DiClemente, 1983) has been used as a foundation for intervention design and its benefit is that it allows an intervention to be tailored to an individual's needs and their specific stage. A further strength of the model is that the individual's current stage can be used as an indicator of success. If we look at the stages of change model when applied to condom use we can explore how we can place individuals within each of the stages (see Figure 7.3).

In this model, women who reported using condoms consistently (i.e. every time they had sex) for at least six months with their main partners were in 'maintenance', those using condoms consistently but for less than six months were in 'action', those who intended to use condoms consistently in the next month were in 'preparation', those who intended to use condoms consistently sometime within the next six months were in 'contemplation', and those who did not intend to use condoms consistently were in 'pre-contemplation'.

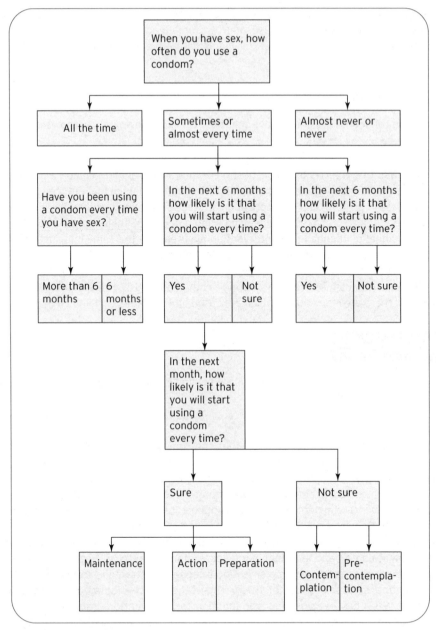

Figure 7.3 Stages of change model applied to condom use
Source: Adapted from Gielen *et al.* (2001)

Applying this to Gary and Debbie

What would you consider Gary and Debbie's current stage of change?

This is one simple way of classifying individuals into stage of change and basing interventions on this assessment. However, there are other, more sophisticated models. Level of motivation to practise safer sex can be reported in a number of ways. For example, asking individuals a set of questions allows them to be categorised into each of the stages (see Table 7.5).

Table 7.5 Allocating individuals to stage of change

Question	Stage of change
Are you basically satisfied with your sexual behaviours and don't want to change them?	Pre-contemplators
Are you thinking about making changes to your sexual behaviour soon (i.e. in the next month)?	Contemplators
Are you going to make changes to your sexual behaviour in the next month?	Preparation
Have you made changes to your sexual behaviour in the past six months?	Action
Have you made changes to your sexual behaviour in the past six months and not returned to the previous pattern?	Maintenance

Alternatively (in a less formal manner), the healthcare professional could simply ask the individual what their sexual behaviour was and whether they intended to change it.

Key message

Assessing an individual's stage of change allows you to tailor appropriate interventions.

According to the SoC model, there are two important factors for predicting movement towards adoption of safer behaviour: self-efficacy and decisional balance. An individual's self-efficacy for performing the behaviour has been shown to have a linear relationship with more movement to safer behaviour. As individuals progress towards maintenance of positive health behaviour, their confidence in their ability to carry out the behaviour increases (see Chapter 4 for fuller discussion on self-efficacy). Decisional balance is simply weighting the perceived pros and cons of behaviour change and how these cognitions about health behaviour relate to stage of change. Typically, people in the pre-contemplation stage identify more cons associated with the behaviour, whereas those in the action or maintenance stages perceive greater pros of engaging in the behaviour. Some of the pros and cons of condom use most frequently reported are presented in Table 7.6.

Discussion point

Presented in Table 7.6 are the pros and cons of condom use. Another way of looking at this is the pros and cons of unprotected sex. Consider what these may be and how they could impact on Gary and Debbie.

Table 7.6 Pros and cons of condom use

Pros	Cons
Protects from STIs	Sensation reduced
Prevents unwanted pregnancy	Interrupts the moment
Reduces mess	Added expense/inconvenience to obtain
Increases female pleasure	Embarrassment when communicating with partner
Lengthens time for intercourse	

Studies have indicated that, not surprisingly, the pros and cons of condom use are consistently the best predictor of progression to and maintenance of consistent condom use. Hence, the message for the healthcare professional is clear: deal with the pros and cons of condom use at the outset. One of the major tasks may be dealing with the negative aspects of condom wear and correcting misconceptions.

Key message

Always deal with the misconceptions of safe sex and condom use.

One way of dealing with the misconceptions is to attempt to reinterpret the use of condom; for example, moving from the condom as 'safety wear' to condoms as 'pleasure promoters' or eroticising the condom. One project, the Pleasure Project (Philpott et al., 2006), aims to promote condoms as sexy and pleasurable and lists a number of 'quick and dirty ways' to illustrate the benefits of condoms. So, for example, opening a male condom packet can be a sign that a person is ready for sex. Carrying condoms in a pocket or handbag when going out, and showing them to a potential partner, can illustrate how interested the person is in sex, while also encouraging condom use (Philpott et al., 2006, p. 25).

For example, Table 7.7 outlines the previously highlighted negatives associated with condom wear and suggests how these can be corrected or addressed.

A second key element derived from the studies exploring the SoC is that interventions need to be tailored to the stage of change. The model suggests that different processes in

Table 7.7 Misconceptions around condom wear

Cons	How
Sensation reduced	Add additional lube which can enhance the experience for both partners
Interrupts the moment	Can add to the moment, as it can signify to the partner that they are ready for sex
Added expense/inconvenience to obtain	Can be obtained free from a number of sources
Embarrassment when communicating with partner	Should be able to embrace the moment and actually can add to the pleasure for both parties

behaviour change, such as raising consciousness and self-reinforcement, are necessary at different stages. Thus, interventions focusing on cognitive and emotional factors will be the most influential in early stages, whereas action-orientated approaches are effective in later stages.

For example, for inconsistent condom users, interventions should first target increasing the advantages of using condoms (e.g. lengthen duration of sexual intercourse, decrease messiness, increase female pleasure) and then promote and model skills for communication with partners about condoms. Maintaining consistent condom use is a challenge and interventions will need to focus on novel ways to sustain interest in the effectiveness and positive aspects of condoms. For individuals who use condoms consistently, interventions might adhere to relapse prevention models whereby the goals are to preserve the positive attitude towards condoms, maintain consistent communication with partners about condoms and reinforce perceptions of vulnerability to STIs.

Key message

There are different interventions dependent on the individual's stage of change.

There is a difference between some of the other behaviours discussed in this book and safer sex: for example, with smoking, diet and exercise, behaviour change is largely an individual choice. The adoption of condom use, however, is a behaviour that often demands communication and agreement between partners. It may necessitate an assessment of one's own risk, and also the risk of one's partner(s). Therefore, communication with partners about condom use and perceived personal vulnerability to STIs and HIV must be taken into account. Furthermore, we must return to our original point: sex is a pleasurable activity and this has to be encouraged with partners and individuals. The fear message will not work.

Key message

It is essential that individuals are empowered to insist on condom use.

Given that attempting to provide safer sex education can be problematic, it is essential that some broad-based messages are promoted and these are provided in Table 7.8. As can be noted, the emphasis is on pleasure rather than fear. It is about promoting the activity in a safe way rather than attempting to scare people into changing.

Key message

Messages for contraceptive method can, and should be, promoted through a variety of routes.

Table 7.8 Tips for sexual health educators

Tip	Comment
Have a realistic attitude	Appreciate that different sexual practices and attitudes are evident
Get advice from the target audience	Pleasure and sexiness are often culturally specific, so tailor the message appropriately
Remain comfortable about talking about sex and pleasure	Trainers and health educators need to be able to talk about sex and pleasure seeking in appropriate language
Focus on pleasure and sex rather than disease	It is important to strike a balance between promoting pleasure and promoting health
Promote positive messages rather than messages of fear or shame	If people are fearful or shamed then they are less likely to request assistance
Focus on the individual issues	Ensure that any counselling/intervention is tailored to deal with the individual concerns and not a predetermined agenda
Be realistic in an assessment of risk	Ensure the individual client assesses their own risks and acceptable measures of risk reduction
Support positive changes	Small steps are positive, and moving from one stage to another can be seen as positive
Clarify misconceptions	Clarify rather than deal with general discussions
Use appropriate language	Ensure that over-technical language is avoided and that the individual feels comfortable when discussing sex

Box 7.2 Applying Research in Practice

Predicting intentions to perform protective sexual behaviours among Norwegian adolescents (Myklestad and Rise, 2008)

This study examined the relative contribution of the Theory of Planned Behaviour (TPB) components in predicting adolescents' intentions to use condoms and contraceptive pills. The extent to which risk-promoting and health-promoting prototypes improved the predictive utility of the TPB was also explored.

A questionnaire was administered to 196 pupils at three schools in Oslo during 2001. The mean age was 14.5 years.

Health risk and normative beliefs, especially partner's opinion, were the most important predictors for boys' condom decisions, while for girls normative and attitudinal considerations were most important. Perceived risk of contracting a sexually transmitted disease was the most important predictor among behavioural beliefs for condom intention for both boys and girls. Normative beliefs, especially parental opinions, were most important for girls' decision to use contraceptive pills.

Results indicated that normative influence was important for both boys' and girls' decisions concerning contraception. Romantic partner was the key individual for boys' condom decisions,

→

whereas girls' contraception decisions were influenced by the opinions of their parents and friends. Effective school interventions may include group discussions, in which misunderstandings concerning friends' opinions towards risky sexual behaviour are clarified. Encouraging parents to communicate their opinions about contraception to their teenage girls may be another effective intervention. Influencing girls' attitudes towards condom use is also recommended, as are interventions in which risk information about the consequences of not using a condom are conveyed.

Conclusion

Sexual behaviour is a natural behaviour that has, at its root, a fundamental physiological purpose. However, it serves a range of other cultural, emotional, psychological and social purposes which have to be considered when attempting to promote safe sexual behaviour. The promotion of a safe sex message is important given the rise in sexually transmitted diseases both nationally and worldwide. Psychological factors contribute to whether people engage in safe sex or not, and social cognitive models have proved successful in predicting condom use. There are a number of key elements from the Stages of Change model that can be used in promoting safe sex.

Summary points

- Researchers generally define sexual behaviour as any behaviour that involves a sexual response of the body; however, individuals (particularly adolescents) will define it differently.
- Safe sex is hard to define but involves taking steps to reduce the chance of contracting or transmitting STIs. Most people associate this with condom use and/or monogamy.
- The UK has seen the largest rise in the number of HIV cases in Western Europe since 2000 and cases of other STIs, such as chlamydia and gonorrhoea, are also increasing.
- Evidence suggests that consistent and correct condom use is associated with reduced STI transmission. Despite this, many people in the UK are not consistently practising safe sex.
- Alcohol and illicit drug use are associated with risky sexual behaviours.
- Social cognition models have been shown to predict some safe sex practices.
- Self-efficacy is a key variable in promoting safe sex.
- Interventions to reduce unsafe sex include providing sex education in schools and mass media campaigns.
- Interventions have been shown to be more effective when they are targeted to specific audiences and are based on psychological theory.
- Individuals can be classified according to their stage of change and this information used to promote condom use.
- Misconceptions about condom use must be addressed and these can be redefined positively.
- Sexual behaviour change is more effective if promoted within a positive pleasure framework.

Putting this into action

Consider Gary and Debbie:

- How would you assess their respective sexual behaviour?
- What sort of problems are Debbie and Gary potentially facing?
- What stage do you think both Gary and Debbie are currently at?
- What do you need to do in order to move Gary into the next stage?
- Develop an action plan for Gary (and discuss how to involve Debbie).

Useful Web links

Condom essential wear 0800 567 123 http://www.condomessentialwear.co.uk/

R U Thinking about sex and 0800 28 29 30 www.ruthinking.co.uk relationships?

Teenage Health Freak www.teenagehealthfreak.org

NHS - sexual health www.nhs.uk/Livewell

References

Abraham, C., Kraché, B., Dominic, R. and Frische, I. (2002). Does research into the social cognitive antecedents of action contribute to health promotion? A content analysis of safe-sex promotion leaflets. *British Journal of Health Psychology*, 7, 227-246.

Ajzen, I. (1985). From intention to actions: A theory of planned behaviour. In J. Kuhl and J. Beckman (eds) Action-Control: From Cognition to Behaviour. Available at (accessed 20 December 2007). http://www.people.umass.edu/aizen/publications.html

Barry, P.M. and Klausner, J.D. (2006). *The Impact of STIs. Clinical Issues*. Accessed 17 December 2007: www.mioonline.com

Barrett, A. (2004). Teens and oral sex: A sexual health educator's perspective. *Canadian Journal of Human Sexuality*, 13, 197-200.

Bartlett, R., Holdtich-Davis, D. and Belyea, M. (2007). Problem behaviour in adolescents. *Pediatric Nursing*, 33, 35-36.

Berer, M. (2006). Condoms, yes! 'Abstinence', no. *Reproductive Health Matters*, 14, 6-16.

Browning, J.R., Hatfield, E., Kessler, D. and Levine, T. (2000). Sexual motives, gender and sexual behaviour. *Archives of Sexual Behavior*, 29, 135-153.

Bruckner, H., and Bearman, P. (2005). After the compromise: The STD consequences. *Canadian Journal of Human Sexuality*, 13, 197-200.

Bryan, A.D., Aitken, L.S. and West, S.G. (1996). Increasing condom use: Evaluation of a theory-based intervention to decrease sexually transmitted disease in women. *Health Psychology*, 15, 371-382.

Bryan, A.D., Aitken, L.S. and West, S.G. (1997). Young women's condom use: The influence of responsibility for sexuality, control over the sexual encounter, and perceived susceptibility to common STDs. *Health Psychology*, 16, 468–479.

Buhi. E.R. and Goodson, P. (2007). Predictors of adolescent and sexual behaviour and intention: A theory-guided systematic review. *Journal of Adolescent Health*, 40(1), 4–21.

Carey, R.F., Herman, W.A., Retta, S.M., Rinaldi, J.ER., German, B.A. and Athey, T.W. (1992). Effectiveness of latex condoms as a barrier to human immunodeficiency virus-sized particles under conditions of simulated use. *Sexually Transmitted Disease*, 19, 230–234.

Chambers, W.C. (2007). Oral sex: Varied behaviours and perceptions in a college population. *Journal of Sex Research*, 44(1), 28–42.

Choi, K.H. and Catania, J.A. (1996). Changes in multiple sexual partnerships, HIV testing and condom use among US heterosexuals 18–49 years of age, 1990 and 1992. *American Journal of Public Health*, 86, 554–556.

Collazo, A.A. (2004). Theory-based predictors of intention to engage in precautionary sexual behaviour among Puerto Rican high school adolescents. *Journal of HIV/AIDS Prevention in Children and Youth*, 6(1), 1–120.

Collins, G. (1985). Impact of AIDS: Patterns of homosexual life changing. *New York Times*, 22 July, p. 84.

Condomessentialwear. (2009). www.condomessentialwear. co.uk (accessed 19 December 2007).

Davis, K.R. and Weller, S.C. (1999). The effectiveness of condoms in reducing heterosexual transmission of HIV. *Family Planning Perspectives*, 31, 272–279.

Dilorio, C., Dudley, W.N., Kelly, M., Soet, J., Mbwara, J. and Sharpe Potter, J. (2001). Social cognitive correlates of sexual experience and condom use among 13 through 15 year old adolescents. *Journal of Adolescent Health*, 29, 208–216.

Dunn, L., Ross, B., Caines, T. and Howorth, P. (1998). A school-based HIV/AIDS prevention education programme: Outcomes of peer-led versus community nurse-led interventions. *Canadian Journal of Human Sexuality*, 7, 339–345.

Evans, D.L. and Tripp, J.H. (2006). Sex education: The case for primary prevention and peer education. *Current Paediatrics*, 16, 95–99.

Fishbein, M. and Ajzen, I. (1975) *Belief, Attitude, Intention and Behaviour: An Introduction to Theory and Research*. London: Addison-Wesley.

Fontes, M. and Roach, P. (2007). Predictors and confounders of unprotected sex: A UK web-based study. *European Journal of Contraception & Reproductive Health Care*, 12(1), 36–45.

Gallo, M.F., Steiner, M.J., Warner, L., Hylton-Kong, T., Figueroa, J.P., Hobbs, M.M. and Behets, F.M. (2007). Self-reported condom use is associated with reduced risk of Chlamydia, gonorrhoea, and trichomoniasis. *Sexually Transmitted Diseases*, 34(10), 829–833.

Gebhardt, W.A., Kuyper, L. and Dusseldorp, E. (2006). Condom use at first intercourse with a new partner in female adolescents and young adults: the role of cognitive planning and motives for having sex. *Archives of Sexual Behavior*, 35(2), 217–223.

Gielen, A.C., Fogarty, L.A., Armstrong, K, Green, B.M., Cabral, R., Milstein, B., Galavotti, C. and Heilig, C.M. (2001). Promoting condom use with main partners: A behavioural intervention trail for women. *AIDS and Behaviour*, 5, 193–204.

Godin, G., Gagnon, H., Lambert, L.D. and Conner, M. (2005). Determinants of condom use among a random sample of single heterosexual adults. *British Journal of Health Psychology*, 10, 85-100.

Guiguet, M., Lepont, F., Retel, O. and Valleron, A.J. (1994). Changes in HIV behavior among French heterosexuals: Patterns of sexual monogamy and condom use between 1988-1991. *Journal of Acquired Immune Deficiency Syndromes*, 7, 1290-1291.

Hahm, H.C., Lahiff, M. and Barreto, R.M. (2006). Asian American adolescents' first sexual intercourse: Gender and acculturation differences. *Perspectives on Sexual and Reproductive Health*, 38(1), 28-36.

Hatherall, B., Ingham, R., Stone, N. and McEachran, J. (2007). How, not just if, condoms are used: The timing of condom application and removal during vaginal sex among young people in England. *Sexually Transmitted Infections*, 83, 68-70.

Holland, J., Ramazanoglu, C., Scott, S. *et al.* (1992). Risk, power, and the possibility of pleasure: Young women, safer sex. AIDS Care, 4, 273-283.

HPA. (2007a). Health Protection Agency. *Statistics - Genital Herpes*. Available at: http://www.hpa.org.uk/infections/topics_az/hiv_and_sti/Stats/STIs/herpes/statistics.htm (accessed 18 December 2007).

HPA. (2007b). Health Protection Agency. *Hepatitis B - General Information*. Available at http://www.hpa.org.uk/infections/topics_az/hepatitis_b/gen_info.htm (accessed 18 December 2007).

HPA. (2007c). Health Protection Agency. *HIV and Other STI's - 2.1 HIV*. Available at http://www.hpa.org.uk/web/HPAweb_C/1203496897276 (accessed 18 December 2007).

HPA. (2008). *All New Episodes Seen at GUM Clinics: 1998-2007. United Kingdom and Country Specific Tables*. London: Health Protection Agency.

Lear, D. (1995). Sexual communication in the age of AIDS: The construction of risk and trust among young adults. *Social Science and Medicine*, 41, 1311-1323.

Lindsey, R. (1985). Bathhouse curbs called help in coast AIDS fight. *New York Times*, 24 October, p. A19.

Logan, T., Cole, J. and Leukefeld, C. (2003). Gender differences in the context of sex exchange among crack users. *AIDS Education and Prevention*, 15(5), 448-464.

Marston, C. and King, E. (2006). Factors that shape people's sexual behaviour: A systematic review. *Lancet*, 368(9547), 1581-1586.

Miller, W.R. and Rollnick, S. (2002). *Motivational Interviewing: Preparing People for Change* (2nd edn). New York: Guilford Press.

Morin, S.F., Charles, K.A. and Malyon, A.K. (1984). The psychological impact of AIDS on gay men. *American Psychologist*, 39, 1288-1293.

Moskowitz, J.M., Assunta Ritieni, A., Tholandi, M. and Xia, M. (2006). How do Californians define safe sex? *Californian Journal of Health Promotion*, 4(1), 109-118.

Myklestad, I. and Rise, J. (2008). Predicting intentions to perform protective sexual behaviours among Norwegian adolescents. *Sex Education*, 8(1), 107-124.

NSOS (2007). *Omnibus Survey Report No. 33 Contraception and Sexual Health 2006/07: A report on research using the National Statistics Omnibus Survey produced on behalf of the*

Information Centre for health and social care. Available at: http://www.statistics. gov.uk/
downloads/theme_health/contraception2006-07.pdf (accessed 7 November 2007).

ONS (2006). *Sexual Health.* http://www.statistics.gov.uk/CCI/nugget.asp?ID=1330&Pos=&
ColRank=2&Rank=224 (accessed 18 December 2007).

Philpott, A., Knerr, W. and Boydell, V. (2006). Pleasure and Prevention: When Good Sex is
Safer Sex. *Reproductive Health Matters,* 14, 23-31.

Prochaska, J.O. and DiClemente, C.C. (1983).Stages and processes of self-change smoking:
Towards an integrative model of change. *Journal of Consulting and Clinical Psychology,* 51,
390-395.

Prochaska, J.O. and DiClemente, C.C. (2002). Transtheoretical therapy: Toward a more integrative model of change. *Psychotherapy: Theory, Research and Practice,* 19, 276-288.

Richters, J. and Song, A. (1999). Australian university students agree with Clinton's definition
of sex. *Britain Medical Journal,* 318, 1011.

Rogers, R.W. (1975). A protection motivation theory of fear appeals and attitude change.
Journal of Psychology, 91, 93-114.

Rosenstock, I. (1990). The Health Belief Model: Explaining health behaviour through
expectancies. In K. Glanz, F.M. Lewis and B.K. Rimmer (eds). *Health Behaviour and Health
Education: Theory, Research and Practice.* San Francisco: Jossey-Bass.

Sanderson, C.A. (2000). The effectiveness of a sexuality education newsletter in influencing
teenagers' knowledge and attitudes about sexual involvement and drug use. *Journal of
Adolescent Research,* 15, 674-681.

Santelli, J.S., Kaiser, J., Hirsch, L. *et al.* (2004). Initiation of sexual intercourse among middle
school adolescents: The influence of psychosocial factors. *Journal of Adolescent Health,*
34, 200-208.

Schaalma, H.P., Abraham, C., Gillmore, M.R. and Kok, G. (2004). Sex education as health promotion: What does it take? *Archives of Sexual Behavior,* 33(3), 259-269.

Sheeran, P., Abraham, C. and Orvell, S. (1999). Psychosocial correlates of heterosexual
condom use: A meta-analysis. *Psychological Bulletin,* 125, 90-132.

Shrier, L.A., Ancheta, R., Goodman, E., Chiou, V.M., Lyden, M.R. and Emans, S.J. (2001).
Randomized controlled trials of safer sex intervention for high-risk adolescent girls.
Archives of paediatrics and Adolescent Medicine, 155, 73-79.

Sieving, R., Eisenberg, M., Pettingell, S. and Skay, C. (2006). Friends' influence on adolescents' first sexual intercourse. *Perspectives on Sexual and Reproductive Health,* 38, 13-19.

Slevin, A.P. and Marvin, C.L. (1987). Safe sex and pregnancy prevention: A guide for
health practitioners working with adolescents. *Journal of Community Health Nursing,* 4,
235-241.

Stone, N., Hatherall, B., Ingham, R. and McEachran, J. (2006). Oral sex and condom use
among young people in the United Kingdom. *Perspectives on Sexual and Reproductive
Health,* 38, 6-12.

Thomas, M.H. (2000). Abstinence-based programs for prevention of adolescent pregnancies:
A review. *Journal of Adolescent Health,* 26, 5-17.

UNAIDS (2006). *UNAIDS/WHO AIDS Epidemic Update: December 2006.* Available at: http://
www.unaids.org/en/HIV_data/epi2006/default.asp (accessed November 2007).

Wald, A., Langenberg, A.G.M., Krantz, E., Douglas, J.M., Handsfield, H.H., DiCarlo, R.P., Adimora, A.A., Izu, A.E., Morrow, R.A. and Corey, C. (2005). The relationship between condom use and herpes simplex virus acquisition. *Annals of Internal Medicine,* 143, 707–713.

Wellings, K., Field, J., Johnson, A.M. and Wadsworth, J. (1994). *Sexual Behaviour in Britain: The National Survey of Sexual Attitudes and Lifestyles*. Harmondsworth: Penguin.

Chapter 8
Stopping illicit drug use

LEARNING OBJECTIVES

At the end of this chapter you will:

- Understand the extent of illegal drug misuse in UK
- Have explored the consequences of illegal drug misuse
- Appreciate the complexity in assessing which factors increase risk of drug taking and which factors are protective against illicit drug use
- Be able to identify various psychological approaches to the prevention and treatment of illicit drug use
- Be able to apply the stages of change model to illicit drug use reduction
- Have explored the concept of harm reduction and relapse prevention

Case study

Ricky is a 20-year-old man who lives with his girlfriend in their shared flat. Currently he is working as a grass cutter for the local council. His parents had high hopes for him as he achieved 11 GCSEs at A* level. However, following this success he became more involved in cannabis (he had previously been involved in glue sniffing and some alcohol abuse) and was eventually expelled from school for attempting to sell cannabis to his peers. Since these early days at school he has always used cannabis, but has also developed a habit for cocaine. Despite his assurances, his girlfriend feels that it does affect both his job and their social life. She has threatened to leave him and has given him a final ultimatum.

He has started acting strangely and is under investigation at work for some bizarre behaviour exhibited recently and for poor time keeping. However, Ricky is finding it hard to deal with the pressures of working regularly and has started to increase his drug intake. Furthermore, he has started selling drugs at a local drug haunt as he is

→

finding it difficult to fund his drug taking on his current salary. He goes down the local pub most nights where he meets his mates before going back to either their flat or his own to take drugs into the early hours. Although this is a habit that Ricky has tried to deal with on a number of occasions, he always seems to be drawn back to the same circle of friends and ends up on a downward spiral. His girlfriend has come to you in tears and wants support and advice – how can she help Ricky?

Discussion point

What would you suggest for Ricky? What do you think are the underlying factors that are promoting and supporting Ricky in his behaviour? What can his girlfriend do? When, and if, Ricky came to see you, what would you recommend? How has Ricky's drug career progressed?

Introduction

There are many forms of illicit drug abuse, and the first thing we must do is explore the various definitions. The criteria for harmful use (ICD-10) and substance misuse (DSM-IV) are presented in Table 8.1. Although this is useful from a formal perspective and allows for an individual's illicit drug use to be objectively quantified, there are several unanswered issues to be resolved. Firstly, it is important to note the difference between *drug use* and *drug abuse*: people who use drugs do not necessarily become continual users and they, in turn, do not necessarily become addicts (Gorusch, 1980). Hence, we should talk about 'use', which refers to any use, including experimentation; 'misuse', referring to problematic or very heavy use; 'addiction', which refers to a chronic relapsing condition characterised by compulsive drug seeking and abuse. Finally, we should make it clear that 'Substance' refers to alcohol, illicit drugs and volatile substances. Since Chapter 5 deals with alcohol, this chapter restricts itself to illicit drugs and volatile substances (i.e. so-called 'glue sniffing').

Key message

It is important to distinguish between misuse, use, abuse and addiction.

Government recommendations

In the UK there are three classes of drugs (A, B, C) that are termed as controlled substances under the Misuse of Drugs Act (1971), with Class A being considered the most harmful (see Table 8.2). Hence, illegal drug misuse is socially constructed – it is those drugs defined by the government to be illegal and the most harmful. Hence, for example, cannabis was until recently (2001) a Class B drug but was then classified as Class C. However, in January 2009 it was reclassified as a Class B drug. Over the period of a decade, the classification of cannabis has changed twice as a consequence of political and social pressures. Two other drugs, alcohol and tobacco, are not defined as illegal drugs currently, although some consider they should be.

Table 8.1 ICD-10 (WHO, 2007a) and DSM-IV (APA, 1994) criteria for harmful use and substance abuse

ICD-10: Criteria for harmful use	DSM-IV: Criteria for substance abuse
A pattern of psychoactive substance abuse that is causing damage to health, either physical or mental. The diagnosis requires that actual damage should have been caused to the mental or physical health of the user. Socially negative consequences and the disapproval of others are not in themselves evidence of harmful use	• Recurrent substance use resulting in a failure to fulfil major role obligations at work, school or home • Recurrent substance abuse in situations in which it is physically hazardous • Recurrent substance-related legal problems • Continued substance use despite having persistent or recurrent social or interpersonal problems caused or exacerbated by the effects of the substance

Applying this to Ricky

How would you classify Ricky? Does he use, misuse or abuse illicit drugs? Has he a drug problem?

Table 8.2 Penalties for possession and dealing

		Possession:	Dealing:
Class A	Ecstasy, LSD, heroin, cocaine, crack, magic mushrooms, amphetamines (if prepared for injection)	Up to seven years in prison or an unlimited fine or both	Up to life in prison or an unlimited fine or both
Class B	Amphetamines, methylphenidate (Ritalin), pholcodine, cannabis	Up to five years in prison or an unlimited fine or both	Up to 14 years in prison or an unlimited fine or both
Class C	Tranquilisers, some painkillers, gamma hydroxybutyrate (GHB), ketamine	Up to two years in prison or an unlimited fine or both	Up to 14 years in prison or an unlimited fine or both

The World Health Organisation (2007b) estimated the extent of worldwide psychoactive substance use to be 2 billion alcohol users (see Chapter 5), 1.3 billion smokers (see Chapter 6) and 185 million drug users (of course, the definition of 'illicit' drugs differs between cultures and countries). As can be noted the major substances used are alcohol and tobacco, with drug use (or substance, more correctly) being a distant third (see Figure 8.1).

Discussion point

Often alcohol, tobacco and drug misuse coexist. For example, Ricky smokes, drinks and takes both cannabis and cocaine. It is likely that his diet and physical activity are also poor. In such situations, which behaviour do you tackle first? The most important or the 'quick fix'? Do you let Ricky decide, or the healthcare professional?

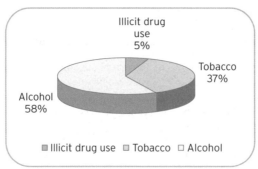

Figure 8.1 World extent of psychoactive substance use
Source: WHO, 2007a

The World Health Organisation (2007b) estimated that the global burden of disease related to tobacco, alcohol and illicit drugs contributed a total of 12.4% of all deaths world-wide in the year 2000.

In terms of the UK, some 10% of the population report having taken illegal drugs in the preceding year (see Table 8.3). People aged between 16 and 24 years are more likely than older people to have used drugs recently and more than a quarter (28%) of all 16–24-year-olds had used at least one illicit drug in the year. The use of Class A drugs in the last year among 16–24-year-olds has remained stable since 1995 and stands around 8% (see Table 8.4). Other figures indicate that over a third of the 16–59-year-old population has 'ever' used an illegal drug, and currently there are estimated to be about four million users of illicit drugs in the UK (Condon and Smith, 2003). The National Treatment Agency for substance misuse (2005) estimates that about 250,000 people in England and Wales will develop serious problems associated with their drug use every year.

Health consequences of illicit drug use

It goes without saying that individuals who take illicit drugs face potentially significant health risks – the drugs taken are often not controlled or supervised by professionals and those that are sold 'on the streets' are of variable quality, strength and origin. As well as the immediate health risks, drugs can also lead to long-term addiction, health damage and potentially death.

Table 8.3 The proportion of 16–59-year-olds reporting to having used drugs in the year 2006/07

Drug	Percentages
Class A	
Any cocaine	2.6
Cocaine powder	2.6
Crack cocaine	0.2
Ecstasy	1.8
Hallucinogens	0.7
LSD	0.2
Magic mushrooms	0.6
Opiates	0.2
Heroin	0.1
Methadone	0.1
Class A/B	
Amphetamines	1.3
Class B/C	
Tranquillisers	0.4
Class C	
Anabolic steroids	0.1
Cannabis	8.2
Ketamine	0.3
Not Classified	
Amyl Nitrite	1.4
Glues	0.2
Total	
Class A	3.4
Any Drug	10.0

Source: Crime in England and Wales 2006/7, 4th edn, Home Office (Nicholas, S., Kershaw, C. and Walker, K. (eds) 2008), © Crown copyright 2008. Reproduced under the terms of the Click-Use Licence

Drug-related deaths often attract a great deal of political and media attention. The Office for National Statistics (ONS) produces mortality statistics for drug-related deaths based upon information on death certificates (see Table 8.5), and these indicate nearly 3,000 deaths related to substance misuse in the UK.

These deaths are, of course, relatively low and significantly less than those caused by either alcohol or smoking (see Chapters 5 and 6). Nonetheless, they are avoidable and significant to individual families and friends. Obviously, the consequences of substance misuse are not restricted to death, and there may be an impact on health that differs dependent on the drugs being used (see Table 8.6). However, what is clear is that all illicit drug use is associated with significant morbidity.

Table 8.4 Estimate of last year drug use in 16–24-year-olds

Drug	Number of users
Cocaine	270,000
Crack	27,000
Ecstasy	312,000
LSD	49,000
Magic mushrooms	99,000
Heroin	12,000
Methadone	9,000
Amphetamines	216,000
Tranquillisers	47,000
Cannabis	1,497,000
Amyl nitrite	247,000
Glues	29,000
Class A	474,000
Any drug	1,629,000

Source: Crime in England and Wales 2006/7, 4th edn, Home Office (Nicholas, S., Kershaw, C. and Walker, K. (eds) 2008), © Crown copyright 2008. Reproduced under the terms of the Click-Use Licence

Table 8.5 Number of UK deaths related to substance misuse (as recorded on death certificate)

Drug	Deaths
Heroin and morphine	842
Methadone	220
Cocaine (including crack)	176
All amphetamines	103
(of which MDMA/ecstasy)	58
Cannabis	19
Gamma-hydroxybutyrate (GHB)	4
All benzodiazepines	190
Zopiclone/Zolpidem	48
Barbiturates	14
All antidepressants	401
Paracetamol (including compound formulations)	466
Codeine (non-compound formulation)	44
Dihydrocodeine (non-compound formulation)	106
Aspirin	19
Tramadol	53
Total	**2763**

Source: Drug-related poisoning deaths: by selected type of drug, 1993 to 2000, Social Trends, 33 ed. (ONS 2005), © Crown Copyright 2005. Reproduced under the terms of the Click-Use Licence

Table 8.6 Illicit drug use and health consequences

Drug	Consequences
Heroin and morphine	Short-term effects include a surge of euphoria followed by alternately wakeful and drowsy states and cloudy mental functioning. Associated with fatal overdose and, particularly in users who inject the drug, infectious diseases such as HIV/AIDS and hepatitis
Cocaine (including crack)	A powerfully addictive drug, cocaine usually makes the user feel euphoric and energetic. Common health effects include heart attacks, respiratory failure, strokes and seizures. Large amounts can cause bizarre and violent behaviour. In rare cases, sudden death can occur on the first use of cocaine or unexpectedly thereafter
Club drugs (the most common club drugs include GHB, Rohypnol, ketamine, methamphetamine)	Chronic use of MDMA may lead to changes in brain function. GHB abuse can cause coma and seizures. High doses of ketamine can cause delirium, amnesia and other problems. Mixed with alcohol, Rohypnol can incapacitate users and cause amnesia
Cannabis	Short-term effects include memory and learning problems, distorted perception, and difficulty thinking and solving problems
LSD	Unpredictable psychological effects. With large enough doses, users experience delusions and visual hallucinations. Physical effects include increased body temperature, heart rate and blood pressure; sleeplessness; and loss of appetite
Ecstasy	Short-term effects include feelings of mental stimulation, emotional warmth, enhanced sensory perception and increased physical energy. Adverse health effects can include nausea, chills, sweating, teeth clenching, muscle cramping and blurred vision
PCP/Phencyclidine	Many PCP users are brought to emergency rooms because of overdose or because of the drug's unpleasant psychological effects. In a hospital or detention setting, people high on PCP often become violent or suicidal

Applying this to Ricky

What healthcare problems is Ricky potentially facing?

Assessment of illicit drug use

There are a number of ways of assessing drug use and misuse. For the non-specialist healthcare professional the most appropriate way of dealing with an individual client or patient who is suspected of misusing illicit drugs is through the Five A's (as discussed in Chapter 6). In short: *Ask, Assess, Advise, Assist and Arrange*. These will be dealt with in this chapter; firstly, what to *ask* and *assess*. The first question that has to be posed is whom to ask (or to screen for drug problems). Although some suggest screening all patients, it is probably more efficient and sensible to use a screening tool with those who you suspect have a problem. Patients should be screened for alcohol, illicit drugs tobacco, misuse of prescription drugs,

Table 8.7 'Red Flag' for substance abuse problems

Complaints	Physical findings
Frequent absence from school or work	Mild tremor
History of trauma or accidents	Smell of alcohol/cannabis or aftershave/
Depression or anxiety	mouthwash (to mask odours)
Labile hypertension	Enlarged, tender liver
GI symptoms (e.g. diarrhoea, weight	Nasal irritation (suggestive of cocaine insufflation)
change)	Conjunctival irritation
Sexual dysfunction	Labile blood pressure, tachycardia
Sleep disorder	Signs of COPD, hepatitis B or C, HIV
	Dilated or constricted pupils
	Track marks or abscesses
	Hallucinations
	Nystagmus
Behaviour patterns	**Laboratory**
Sedation	Elevated MCH, GGT, SGOT
Inebriation	Anaemia
Euphoria	Positive urine toxicology for drugs
Agitation	
Disorientation	
Prescription drug seeking behaviour	
Suicidal ideations/attempts	

and other substances when they present with some key 'red flag' symptoms (see Table 8.7) as these are the ones that probably need most careful attention (Mersy, 2003).

Key message

Look out for red flags before screening for substance misuse.

Applying this to Ricky

On the basis of the case study, what red flags are there? Would you screen him?

The assessment should be performed by the healthcare professional or other staff member who has an ongoing relationship with the patient. Given the importance of the family in the development and maintenance of drug use, it is always useful to include family members in questions about drug use.

The most effective way of assessing a potential client is through an interview (or self-administered tool). Although several such questionnaires are available, the CAGE question-naire (Ewing, 1984) is the most practical for healthcare professionals to use as a screening tool. CAGE is a mnemonic that asks about attempts to **C**ut down on drinking, **A**nnoyance with criticisms about drinking, **G**uilt about drinking, and using alcohol as an **E**ye-opener.

The CAGE questionnaire consists of 4 questions that probe the respondent's *own feelings* regarding their drinking habits to make a diagnosis. The health practitioner asks the respondent if they have ever *felt* that they should cut down on the amount they regularly drink, or been annoyed by other people's criticisms of their drinking habits, or felt guilty about how much they drink or have felt the need to have a drink first thing in the morning to face the day. Each question carries a score of '0' for 'no' and '1' for 'yes' as an answer. A total score of '2' or more is considered clinically significant and worthy of further investigation.

Although initially designed for alcohol (as you can tell), it has been adapted for use with other drugs (see Table 8.8). The questionnaire takes approximately one minute to complete and can act as a screening tool to ensure that the healthcare professional is prompted to look further.

Table 8.8 CAGE questions Adapted to Include Drugs (CAGE-AID)

1. Have you ever felt you ought to cut down on your drinking or drug use?
2. Have people annoyed you by criticising your drinking or drug use?
3. Have you felt bad or guilty about your drinking or drug use?
4. Have you ever had a drink or used drugs first thing in the morning to steady your nerves or to get rid of a hangover (eye-opener)?

Source: Brown and Rounds (1995)

The normal cut-off for the CAGE is two positive answers, although if one is positively responded to then this may suggest the healthcare professional should look further.

The CAGE questionnaire does not differentiate between current and former problems, and it is more accurate in detecting alcoholism than problem drinking. However, it is reported as being 60–90% sensitive when two or more questions are positive and 40–60% specific for excluding substance abuse (Mersy, 2003).

An even shorter questionnaire (if you should need one) is the conjoint screening test that involves only two questions:

- 'In the past year, have you ever drunk or used drugs more than you meant to?' and
- 'Have you felt you wanted or needed to cut down on your drinking or drug use in the past year?' (Brown et al., 2001).
- At least one positive response detects current substance use disorders with nearly 80% sensitivity and specificity.

If the patient denies use, you can acknowledge the wise choice that they have made by abstaining from drugs. However, it is necessary to continue to screen, ideally at each encounter. In some situations, patients may deny use, but a constellation of signs and symptoms suggests abuse. In this case, it may be prudent to re-screen frequently or conduct specific blood/urine/hair testing.

> ## Discussion point
>
> What scores would Ricky get on the CAGE-AID and the conjoint questions? How could you follow this up with his girlfriend? Or with lab testing? If the person (i.e. Ricky) denies they have a problem, what actions can you take?

Why do people take illicit drugs?

There have been a large number of studies that have explored the risk factors associated with drug use. Although there is no 'definitive list' of agreed risk factors supported by conclusive research evidence, there is general agreement that there is no single factor and that the origin of substance misuse is multi-factorial. Various psychosocial factors have been identified as significant correlates of substance use and these can vary across the lifespan (see Table 8.10 later). These factors range from the prenatal environment (including maternal behaviours) through to genetic factors and to wider social influences, including school and socio-economic issues.

> ## Key message
>
> Psychosocial variables are risk variables for illicit drug use.

The role of psychological factors as potential risk factors has been widely studied. For example, Sareen *et al.* (2006) report that anxiety is related to lifetime heroin use and Boden *et al.* (2006) report on the importance of social interaction with substance-using peers and conduct problems in adolescence in the development of illicit drug use. They also report the importance of appreciating other lifestyle behaviours such as cigarette smoking and alcohol consumption, indicating the importance of the interplay and clustering of lifestyle behaviours. Finally, they suggest that risk-taking and novelty-seeking behaviours also have a role. Obviously, there is a need to distinguish between user, abuser and addict (Spooner, 1999) and individual aetiological factors may differ between these groups.

> ## Applying this to Ricky
>
> What risk factors does Ricky have?

The most recent British review was sponsored by the Home Office (Frischer *et al.*, 2004), that report a systematic review of the factors associated with illicit drug initiation (see Table 8.10). This study demonstrated that the factors are considerable, extensive and include both individual elements – e.g. genetics – and more diverse and socially constructed elements – e.g. socio-economic status. What has to be stressed, however, is that these risk factors are

Table 8.9 Factors associated with illicit drug use

Risk factor	Example
Personal factors	Gender
	Age
	Ethnicity
	Life events
	Self-esteem
	Hedonism
	Depression/anxiety
	Mental health factors
	Learning disabilities
	Genetic
Personal factors – behavioural or attitudinal	Early onset of substance use
	Other substance use
	Perceptions of substance use
Interpersonal relationships	Young parents
	Large families
	Parental divorce
	Low discipline
	Family cohesion
	Parental monitoring
	Family substance abuse/psychiatric conditions
	Peer behaviour and use
Structural-environmental and economic	Socio-economic
	Education, school performance and school management
	Drug availability

Source: Adapted from *Estimating the prevalence of problematic and injecting drug use for Drug Action Team areas in England: a feasibility study using the Multiple Indicator Method.* Home Office online report 34/04, available at http://www.homeoffice.gov.uk/rds/pdfs04/rdsolr2404.pdf, Home Office (Frischer, M., Heatlie, H. and Hickman, M. 2004), © Crown copyright 2009. Reproduced under the terms of the Click-Use Licence

not discrete entities but tend to interact, and that these complex interactions are difficult to analyse and comprehend.

A further complication can be added to the already complex picture. Although the factors outlined in Table 8.9 are extensive and interactive, they vary in importance at different ages. As an example of this, Table 8.10 denotes some of the potential risk factors and their importance dependent on the age of the individual concerned.

Key message

Different risk factors are important at different time periods.

Table 8.10 Risk factors for illicit drug use among young people

	Explanation	Prenatal	Birth	0-2 years	3-8 years	9-11 years	12-18 years	Adult
Prenatal environment	Maternal smoking, maternal drug use	✓	✓					
Genetic	Genetic relationship	✓	✓	✓	✓	✓	✓	✓
Family	Parental discipline, family cohesion, parental substance use, parental monitoring, sibling drug use, early life trauma			✓	✓	✓		
School	Truancy, educational attainment, problems at school, school rules				✓	✓	✓	
Friends	Friends' drug use, friends antisocial behaviour						✓	
Psychological traits	Low self-esteem, hedonism, ADHD, phobia, depression, anxiety, aggressive behaviour					✓	✓	
Psychological explanation	Get intoxicated, escape from negative moods						✓	
Socio-economic	Low household income, lack of neighbourhood amenities							✓
Early use of other drugs	Gateway hypothesis						✓	✓
Protective factors								✓

In contrast to these risk factors, research has also identified factors that may protect against drug use. In order to address any illicit drug use, it is important to consider these two factors: the *risk* factors and the *protective* factors.

Key message

When attempting to develop an intervention it is important to consider both the risk factors and the protective factors.

A pure risk factor approach has, as its aim, eliminating, reducing or mitigating risk factors. In contrast, a resiliency approach emphasises prevention by enhancing behavioural factors that protect against vulnerability. Taken together, this approach suggests that both risk factors and vulnerability significantly contribute to a model of adolescent drug use.

Key message

Risk factors have to be taken into account with protective factors.

A number of protective variables have been identified and psychological protective factors in particular are important in shaping the design and implementation of drug protection methods. Specifically, such programmes should highlight that some individuals, despite being exposed to a social environment where drugs are present, as are other risk factors, decide not to use drugs.

Applying this to Ricky

What elements in Ricky's life could be considered protective? How can these be strengthened?

The results of such investigations suggest that the key protective factors include:

- lifestyle aspirations and relationships (other people's disapproval, legal consequences, role as parent, career aspirations);
- practicalities of being a user (availability of time, financial cost);
- physical and psychological consequences of drugs (personal experience with drugs, current health conditions, fear of effect on health, fear of addiction, fear of losing control);
- perceived benefit of using drugs (sources of 'buzz', sources of support/coping mechanism).

The summary of factors that young people identified as facilitating or impeding resilience to drug use is presented in Table 8.11.

Dillon et al. (2007) also explored the youngsters' strategies for avoiding or refusing drugs and suggested that there were two broad types:

- active refusal strategies, saying no;
- avoidance-based refusal strategies.

In refusing offers of drugs, young people want to minimise the risk of repercussions from their refusals, for example damaging friendships or causing arguments or fights. If possible, they do not want to offend the person making the offer, at times emphasising that they respected other people's decisions to use drugs while hoping they in turn would respect their decision not to use. Being confident about their decision not to use and the context in which the offer was made, supported by the people they were with, and feeling able to deal with the threats in terms of the consequences a refusal would have, all facilitated an easier refusal process.

Discussion point

How would you encourage youngsters to refuse drugs but maintain peer friendships?

Table 8.11 Factors associated with resilience to drug use

Other people's motivation to use	Contextual risk factors	Factors making it easier/more difficult to refuse offers	Motivations not to use
• Following example of others • To fit in • Peer pressure • Alleviate boredom • The buzz • Curiosity about effects • Escape problems • Ease physical pain • To look hard • To feel more confident	• In trouble with the police/school • Alcohol use • Boredom • Familial substance use • Mental health issues • Problematic family relationships	• Reputation as resilient to drug use • Type of drug offered • Reputation as a smoker or drinker • Age • Happy to be the odd one out • Being drunk • Offered by friends or strangers	• Other people's disapproval • Fear of effect on health • Fear of addiction • Alternative sources of support/coping mechanisms • Current health conditions • Fear of losing control • Career aspirations • Role as a parent • Availability of time • Financial cost • Personal experience with drugs

Source: Risk, protective factors and resilience to drug use: identifying resilient young people and learning from their experience, Home Office (Dillon, L., Chivite-Matthews, N., Grewal, I., Brown, R., Webster, S., Weddell, E., Brown, G. and Smith, N. (2007)) Home Office, © Crown copyright 2007. Reproduced under the terms of the Click-Use Licence

Applying this to Ricky

What protective factors against illicit drug use does Ricky have?

Box 8.1 Applying research in practice

Cannabis use in adolescents: the impact of risk and protective factors and social functioning (Best *et al.*, 2005)

This study used a school-based sample of 2078 14–16-year-olds from 7 secondary schools in south London to test the social and familial risks and protective factors relating to cannabis use.

Of those surveyed, 40% had been offered cannabis at some point in their lifetime, with an average age of first offer of 13 years. Twenty-four per cent of students reported having ever used cannabis, with 15% having done so during the month prior to assessment.

Those who had used cannabis were more likely than non-users to report lifetime experience of using all other drugs. They were also likely to spend less time regularly with both parents and more time with friends involved in smoking, drinking, drug use and crime.

Among those who had ever used cannabis, frequency of cannabis use was predicted by earlier initiation of drinking and cannabis use, more time spent with drug-using friends and less time spent with the mother. Similarly, among current cannabis users time spent with drug-using friends and cannabis onset age were both significant predictors. Time spent with mother was borderline significant.

Key message

Social factors have a key role in risk and protective factors in the initiation and continued use of cannabis among adolescents.

An implicit, and often explicit, explanation for the resilience shown by individuals is that they show an effective sense of self-efficacy. As previously discussed (see Chapter 4), self-efficacy can be conceptualised as people's beliefs about their capabilities and their ability to put their decisions into practice (Bandura, 1977, 1986). There is a strong relationship between self-efficacy, assertiveness and problem-solving skills, and studies have indicated that young people use a range of strategies to refuse drugs (Epstein et al., 2007). At the same time, effective rational problem-solving skills are also required; for example, balancing the benefits of refusing drugs (e.g. health, finances) with the need to maintain friendships and the negative consequences that may occur as a result of refusal. Consequently, individuals reported that they were the 'odd one out' but were the 'bigger person for saying no'. Hence, success was measured in two ways: continuing to refuse drugs but not compromising their friendships or relationships. Again, the link to self-efficacy is seen in such individuals: the strength of well-being and mastery is increased with such a position.

Key message

Strong self-efficacy is important in being able to refuse offers of drugs from peers, whilst still retaining friendships.

Self-efficacy can be increased through various methods, including verbal persuasion, behavioural rehearsal and actual accomplishment. A sense of personal competency is increased by experiences of progressive mastery or goal attainment. Actions associated with positive internal and external experiences usually are repeated, whereas those associated with negative experiences are discontinued (Bandura, 1986).

Applying this to Ricky

Ricky's self-efficacy could be improved by getting him to achieve personal goals that are small steps towards overall success.

Indeed, enhancing self-efficacy is part of ensuring that youngsters do not start taking drugs and also prevents relapse (Marlatt and Gordon, 1985). Relapse prevention interventions assist in the acquisition and practice of effective coping strategies (both behavioural and cognitive) for managing high-risk situations to enhance self-efficacy when faced with such situations and will be discussed later in this chapter.

Another important factor in the potential initiation of taking illicit drugs is the family, and there are numerous studies that attest to the importance of this unit. The majority of studies have highlighted the strength of parental influence (via both behaviour and attitudes) on young people commencing substance use. Social factors that affect early development within the family, such as a chaotic home environment, ineffective parenting and lack of mutual attachment, have been shown to be crucially important indicators of risk of illicit drug taking (NIDA, 1997).

Velleman et al. (1999) have argued that there are seven areas in which the family context could influence the child's substance use behaviour:

- family relations versus structure;
- family cohesion;
- family communication;
- parental modelling of behaviour;
- family management;
- parental supervision;
- parent/peer influences.

In a comprehensive review Velleman et al. (2005) conclude that: 'There is considerable evidence that family factors are important in increasing risk and also in protecting young people in relation to their taking up of the use of various substances, and in the development in some of those young people of problematic substance use' (p. 103).

Key message

The family and peers have a significant role to play in the development of illicit drug use.

Marijuana use and the gateway hypothesis

One aspect of concern has been the contention that cannabis acts as a 'gateway drug' which leads to the use of other 'harder' drugs such as cocaine, methamphetamine and heroin at a later time (e.g. Kandel, 2003). The gateway hypothesis assumes that there is a link between cannabis use and the onset of other illicit drug use and that the use of cannabis increases the likelihood of using other illicit drugs. Three explanations are often suggested for these patterns: (i) that users of cannabis are more likely to use other illicit drugs because they obtain cannabis from the same black market and hence have more opportunities to use other illicit drugs; (ii) that those who use cannabis at an early age are more likely for other reasons to use other illicit drugs; and (iii) that the pharmacological effects of cannabis increase an adolescent's propensity to use other illicit drugs. Each of these hypotheses has been explored and reviewed, yet there still remains a lack of clarity.

Applying this to Ricky

Does the gateway hypothesis apply to Ricky?

Interventions to reduce illicit drug use

The government's strategy is to reduce the harm that drugs cause by persuading potential users not to use drugs – prevention is better than cure. Consequently, the strategy is aimed at reducing the prevalence of drugs on our streets and reducing the number of current drug users by the use of effective treatments.

Psychological models and illicit drug misuse

The Theory of Planned Behaviour (TBP) and Theory of Reasoned Action (TRA) have been applied to the use of illicit drugs, as have other such models. The Theory of Reasoned Action proposes that an individual's substance abuse behaviours are based on intentions, which in turn are determined by attitudes and perceived social norms regarding substance use (see Chapter 1). Furthermore, the TRA suggests that attitudes are determined by perceived costs and benefits and the affective value placed on those consequences (Petraitis et al., 1995). Intervention campaigns that have targeted key TRA variables have proven successful in preventing substance use (Flynn et al., 1994). On this basis, media campaigns have been developed that influence attitudes and perceived norms regarding substance misuse.

Applying this to Ricky

In order to address Ricky's behaviour there would be a need to influence the attitudes of both himself and his friends.

Such approaches have used psychological models in a social marketing context and it is worth exploring the social marketing techniques that have been used for illicit drug taking. Social marketing is the application of commercial sector marketing tools to the resolution of a number of social and health problems. The idea dates back to 1951 when Wiebe asked the question 'Can brotherhood be sold like soap?' (Wiebe, 1951/1952). Social marketing thinking is now located at the centre of many government health improvement programmes, including reducing illicit drug use. A distinguishing feature of social marketing is that it goes beyond mere education and awareness raising and focuses instead on behaviour. Although outcomes have traditionally been conceptualised in terms of behaviour change, more recent work has expanded this conceptualisation to include the prevention of certain behaviours such as the use of illicit substances (Andreasen, 2006).

The UK's attempt at reducing drug taking through social marketing is 'Project FRANK' which has been widely advertised both through traditional media and using the more informal advanced methods preferred by the target audience (i.e. teenagers). The state of evaluation of such prevention programmes is currently 'very poor' (McGrath et al., 2006). Although no formal evaluation of the FRANK programme's effectiveness of drug reduction has been published, Sumnall and Bellis (2007) suggest that it may be little different from the other social marketing campaigns in the US and UK.

Moreover, Sumnall and Bellis (2007) suggest that such campaigns may have a negative impact on health. They imply that since the campaigns regularly suggest that taking cannabis results in mental health difficulties and affect the 'brain' or 'mind' (see Table 8.6), individuals may begin to believe that they are experiencing such effects. Consequently, Sumnall and Bellis (2007) suggest that cannabis users may suffer 'amotivation, memory loss or even paranoia, not as a direct result of the drug, but through psychological mechanisms induced through high-profile social-marketing campaigns that effectively "sell" such negative effects'. Although there is no clear evidence of such at the moment, it is obviously important for policy makers and healthcare professionals to be aware of such concerns so that they can deal appropriately with any such cases on an individual basis.

On an individual basis, if a patient has shared with you that they are abusing illicit drugs (after you have *Asked* them) but are not ready to take the next step of comprehensive assessment and treatment through a professional programme, then it is useful to turn to the Stages of Change model (SoC) developed by Prochaska *et al.* (1992). As discussed in previous chapters (for example, how the SoC can be applied to smoking interventions in Chapter 6), the five stages of change can be used to guide both the patient and the practitioner and these will be discussed in the intervention section after we have first explored why people actually take drugs. It is useful in both the *Assessment* and the *Advise* section. Although this model has been discussed extensively elsewhere in this chapter, it is worth re-capping this and demonstrating how it can be applied to drug misuse:

1. *Pre-contemplation:* The patient is not considering change during the pre-contemplation stage.
   - They do not believe it is necessary.
   - They do not know or understand the risks involved.
   - They have tried many times to quit without success, so they give up and don't want to try again.
   - They have gone through withdrawal before and are fearful of the process or effects on their body.
   - They feel strongly that no one is going to tell them what to do with their body.
   - They have a mental illness and do not have a good grasp of what using drugs and alcohol means, even when information is given to them.
   - They have family members or partners whom they depend on who use. They may not contemplate changing when everyone else continues to use.

   The individual in pre-contemplation may present as resistant, reluctant, resigned or rationalising.

Presents as:	What the patient is saying:	Healthcare professional response:
Resistant	Don't tell me what to do	Work with the resistance. Avoid confrontation by giving facts about what drugs and alcohol will do to them. Ask what they know about the effects; ask permission to share what you know, and then ask their opinion of the information. This often leads to a reduced level of resistance and allows for a more open dialogue

→

Presents as:	What the patient is saying:	Healthcare professional response:
Reluctant	I don't want to change; there are reasons	Empathise with the real or possible results of changing (for example, if their partner left). It is possible to give strong medical advice to change and still be empathetic to possible negative outcomes to changing. Guide them to problem-solving
Resigned	I can't change, I've tried	Instil hope and explore barriers to change. Increase self-efficacy and confidence. Provide small steps with achievable goals
Rationalising	I don't use that much	Decrease discussion. Listen rather than responding to the rationalisation. Respond to them by empathising and reframing their comments to address the conflict of wanting to be healthy and not knowing whether 'using' is really causing harm

2. *Contemplation:* The patient is ambivalent about changing their behaviour. They can think of the positive reasons to change but are also very aware of the negative sides of change. In this stage it is important to provide the health benefits of changing their behaviour (as discussed earlier in the chapter). There is a need to help the patient explore goals for health, and problem-solve how to deal with the negative aspects of abstinence.

3. *Preparation:* They are exploring options to assist their process of change. They may be experimenting by cutting down or have been able to quit for one or more days. Although their ambivalence is lessening, it is still present and may increase when they are challenged by those around them, triggered by the environment, or are under other types of stress they have handled by using in the past. The healthcare professional should be acknowledging the individual's strengths in reaching this stage but at the same time anticipate problems and pitfalls to changing, and assist the patient in generating their own plan for obtaining abstinence. Problem-solve with them regarding barriers to success.

4. *Action:* The patient has stopped using drugs and/or alcohol and their success needs to be celebrated. Offer to be available for assistance if they feel that they want to use drugs/alcohol again.

5. *Relapse:* Relapse is common and should not be thought of as failure, but as part of the recovery process. At this stage the healthcare professional needs to discuss triggers, stressors and social pressures that may lead to relapse and help the patient plan for them. At future visits, if relapse has occurred, guide the patient towards identifying what steps they used to quit before. Offer hope and encouragement, and allow the patient to explore the negative side of quitting and what they can do to deal with those issues. Offer to help find resources to help the patient return to abstinence.

Applying this to Ricky

What stage is Ricky at? What methods would you adopt to progress him through the stages of change?

One of the most important things that an individual healthcare professional can do for somebody who is abusing drugs is to provide some information and education. Although it is a safe assumption that most individuals will have some knowledge of the effects of alcohol and other drugs, it is important to assess this. Ask the patient what they know and then fill in the missing pieces and clarify misconceptions. This is an excellent opportunity to educate the patient about adverse effects of alcohol/drugs and the benefits of stopping use at any time.

Clinical approaches

If an individual is addicted to illicit drugs or is suffering from alcoholism, there are many professional services available and it is best to refer on for specialist help. At this stage you will be *Assisting* and *Arranging*. It is important at this stage to discuss the benefits of treatment and offer to provide the patient with a referral to a local treatment centre. If the patient is unwilling to make that commitment, ask if they would like some information to take with them if they should change their mind. Schedule the next visit, continue to maintain interest in their progress, and support their efforts in changing.

It is important to discuss the possible strategies for them to stop; for example, individual counselling, 12-step programmes, and other treatment programme. Studies have shown that people given choices are more successful in treatment. Many of these treatments may be medical in nature, but there are a number of psychological approaches to the assessing and preventing of substance misuse and treating people with such problems. A summary of the psychological interventions are presented in Table 8.12. Many approaches are cognitive, behavioural or a mixture of the two in origin.

A number of such cognitive behavioural approaches have developed an evidence base for treating substance misuse and these include interventions such as those described in further detail below.

Contingency management therapies

Contingency management is one form of behavioural therapy in which patients receive incentives for achieving specific behavioural goals. These approaches are based on operant conditioning whereby appropriate behaviour is rewarded with positive consequences and therefore more likely to be repeated. These forms of intervention have particularly strong and robust empirical support. For example, allowing a patient the privilege of taking home methadone doses, contingent on the patient's providing drug-free urine specimens, is associated with significant reductions in illicit drug use (Stitzer *et al.*, 1992). Similarly, Budney *et al.* (1998) demonstrated the efficacy of vouchers redeemable for goods and services, contingent on the patient's providing cocaine-free urine specimens, in reducing targeted drug use and enhancing retention in treatment.

Table 8.12 A brief summary of the main psychological therapies used in treating substance misuse

Behavioural therapy (BT)	A structured therapy focusing on changing behaviour and the environmental factors that trigger maladaptive behaviour. *Includes:*
● **Cue exposure treatment (CET)**	A structured treatment involving exposure to drug-related cues that have been associated with past drug use without consumption of the drug. This is intended to lead to a reduction (or habituation) of reactivity to drug cues and hence to a reduced likelihood of relapse
● **Community reinforcement approach (CRA)**	A behavioural approach that focuses on what the client finds rewarding in their social, occupational and recreational life. It aims to help them change their lifestyle and social environment to support long-term changes in behaviour whereby using substances is less rewarding than not using them
● **Contingency management (CM)**	Also known as voucher-based therapy, this aims to encourage adaptive behaviour by rewarding the client for attaining agreed goals (e.g. no use of illicit drugs as checked by urine screens) and not rewarding them when these goals are unmet (e.g. illicit drug use). Vouchers can usually be exchanged for consumer goods
Cognitive therapy (CT)	A structured therapy using cognitive techniques (e.g. challenging a person's negative thoughts) and behavioural techniques (e.g. behavioural experiments; activity planning) to change maladaptive thoughts and beliefs. *Includes:*
● **Cognitive behavioural therapy (CBT)**	A combination of both cognitive and behavioural therapies
● **Relapse prevention (RP)**	Uses several CBT strategies to enhance the client's self-control and prevent relapse. It highlights problems that the client may face and develops strategies they can use to deal with high-risk situations
Motivational interviewing (MI)	A focused approach aiming to enhance motivation for changing substance use by exploring and resolving the individual's ambivalence about change
Motivational enhancement therapy (MET)	A brief intervention based on MI which also incorporates a 'check-up' assessment and feedback
Twelve-step approaches	Interventions used by self-help organisations like Alcoholics Anonymous. They are based on a philosophy that adopts an illness model and sees substance use as stemming from an innate vulnerability. An individual must acknowledge their addiction and the harm it has caused to themselves and others; they must also accept their lack of control over use and thus the only acceptable goal is abstinence
Other approaches	The involvement of partners and family through marital and family therapy builds on the known social context of substance use. There are also various forms of counselling, group therapy and milieu therapy

There are, of course, some limitations to contingency management interventions. For example, the effects of the intervention tend to reduce after the contingencies are reduced. Secondly, there are costs involved and sometimes these are an impediment to their introduction (Crowley, 1999). Finally, not all users of illicit drugs are responsive to contingency management and there is consequently a need to explore individual differences in responses to behavioural treatment (Carroll and Onken, 2005).

Cognitive behaviour and skills training therapies

Cognitive behaviour approaches, such as relapse prevention, are grounded in social learning theories and principles of operant conditioning. A number of meta-analyses and literature reviews have established the value of cognitive behavioural approaches in drug-using populations (e.g. Irvin et al., 1999). Indeed, several research studies have indicated that CBT is demonstrably effective in the treatment of cocaine-dependent outpatients (e.g. Rohsenow et al., 2000). Another study involving 450 marijuana-dependent individuals demonstrated that a nine-session individual approach that integrated cognitive behaviour therapy and motivational interviewing was more effective than a two-session motivational interviewing approach, which was in turn more effective than a delayed-treatment control condition (MTP Research Group, 2004).

Box 8.2 Applying research in practice

A systematic review of cognitive and behavioural therapies for methamphetamine dependence (Lee and Rawson, 2008)

This paper describes a systematic review of cognitive behavioural and behavioural interventions for methamphetamine users. The review of published literature was undertaken focusing solely on randomised trials.

There were a relatively small number of intervention studies that compared cognitive behavioural or behavioural interventions using randomised trial methodology. Most commonly, studies examined cognitive behaviour therapy (CBT) and/or contingency management (CM). Treatment with CBT appears to be associated with reductions in methamphetamine use and other positive changes, even over very short periods of treatment. CM studies found a significant reduction of methamphetamine use during application of the procedure, but it is not clear if these gains are sustained post-treatment follow-up.

Key message

Based on the studies reviewed, methamphetamine use appears to be reactive to intervention. CBT and CM are two accessible interventions that can be implemented easily within the drug and alcohol services.

Motivational interviewing

Motivational interviewing approaches have strong empirical support for use in treating alcohol users and smokers (see Chapters 5 and 6), with several studies showing significant and durable effects (Dunn et al., 2001; Burke et al., 2003). Marijuana-dependent adults who received motivational interviewing had significant reductions in marijuana use, compared to a delayed-treatment control group (Stephens et al., 2000). However, the research has not always been positive and equivocal results have been found. For example, Miller et al. (2003) did not support the efficacy of motivational interviewing.

Couples and family treatments

The defining feature of couples and family treatments is that they treat drug-using individuals in the context of family and social systems in which substance use may develop or be maintained. The engagement of the individual's social networks in treatment can be a powerful predictor of change, and thus the inclusion of family members in treatment may be helpful in reducing attrition (particularly among adolescents) and addressing multiple problem areas (Liddle *et al.*, 2001). Reviews of such treatments, including meta-analyses, have indicated that these approaches are effective (e.g. Deas and Thomas, 2001).

The National Institute for Health and Clinical Excellence (NICE, 2007) issued guidelines on psychosocial interventions for drug misuse. They made recommendations for the use of psychosocial interventions in the treatment of people who misuse opioids, stimulants and cannabis in the healthcare and criminal justice systems. There were several key priorities for implementation:

- *Brief interventions:* Opportunistic brief interventions focused on motivation should be offered to people in limited contact with drug services (for example, those attending a needle and syringe exchange or primary care settings) if concerns about drug misuse are identified by the service user or staff member.
- *Self-help:* Staff should routinely provide people who misuse drugs with information about self-help groups. These groups should normally be based on 12-step principles.
- *Contingency management:* Drug services should introduce contingency management programmes. The programme should offer incentives (usually vouchers that can be exchanged for goods or services of the service user's choice, or privileges such as take-home methadone doses) contingent on each presentation of a drug-negative test (for example, free from cocaine or non-prescribed opioids).
- *Contingency management to improve physical healthcare:* For people at risk of physical health problems (including transmittable diseases) resulting from their drug misuse, material incentives (for example, shopping vouchers of up to £10 in value) should be considered to encourage harm reduction.

When abstinence is not possible, harm reduction assists a patient to take steps to reduce use and harm to themselves. Strategies for preventing further harm may include:

- Evaluate and refer for underlying problems.
- Encourage the patient to keep track of substance use.
- Decrease use:
  - Reduce dosage and frequency of use.
  - Recommend reducing their use by one-half each day; if this is not possible, any decrease in use is beneficial.
  - Intersperse use with periods of abstinence.
  - Use a safer route of drug administration.
  - Find a substitute for the substance.
- Avoid friends who use.

Whichever method is used, it is important to be constantly vigilant to ensure there is no relapse. Relapse prevention, as previously discussed, is often based on psychological principles

(Marlatt and Donovan, 2005). Relapse prevention is a treatment intervention designed to teach clients a wide range of cognitive and behavioural coping skills to avoid or deal with a brief return to substance use (lapse), or a protracted return to previous levels of use (relapse), following a period of moderation or abstinence.

Marlatt's model of relapse prevention is the model most commonly cited and is supported by considerable literature and research evidence (e.g. Marlatt and Donovan, 2005; Marlatt and Gordon, 1985). In this conceptualisation, relapse is viewed as a process that takes place over time instead of an isolated event. There are several high-risk situations that can alert people to potential problems, and the key is to recognise these situations and do something about them.

High-risk situations involve certain people, places, emotions and thoughts that lead towards a lapse/relapse. In addition, there are several factors occurring outside of high-risk situations that influence a person's chances of success. These include destructive thinking patterns, lifestyle imbalance and a lack of planning. These combined factors can weaken a person's resolve even before he or she faces a high-risk situation.

Marlatt categorised high-risk situations in five key areas: 1. Negative emotional states; 2. Interpersonal conflict; 3. Social pressure; 4. Positive emotional states; and 5. Coping levels. The first three high-risk situations (i.e. negative emotions, interpersonal conflict and social pressure) account for 75% of all relapses (Marlatt and Gordon, 1985). Positive emotional states and coping account for the remaining 25% of all relapses.

In a treatment setting, the client is taught about relapse as a process, including the consequences of using effective rather than ineffective coping strategies. The client is taught how to develop a relapse prevention plan that is tailored to his or her own needs and is shown how to avoid or cope with each specific high-risk situation by using cognitive (e.g. problem solving, challenging distorted thinking, and replacing destructive thoughts with productive thoughts) and behavioural (e.g. social skills, relaxation, assertiveness, pro-social modelling, and functional analysis) coping skills.

In these programmes there is an emphasis on the development of coping strategies. So, for example, at the outset an individual could be asked to highlight their:

Early warning signs   Thoughts and feelings   Coping strategies

Furthermore, they would be asked to write down their high-risk situations, again with their coping strategies. Some examples of triggers and potential coping strategies are provided in Table 8.13. These are based on a cognitive behavioural framework to ensure that the individual thinks positively about their situation and effective ways of dealing with the temptations that may arise.

Table 8.13 Examples of triggers and coping strategies for reducing relapse.

Triggers	Coping strategies
People	Tell them you are busy or otherwise occupied
Places	Go with a friend that does not use drugs or avoid the place
Thoughts	Remember your successes and look at photos reminding you of the good times
Feelings	Listen to music or talk to friends/healthcarepractitioner
Situations	Learn specific coping strategies

Conclusion

Illicit drug use is a behaviour that is, in comparison to the other negative health behaviours discussed in this text, relatively rare. However, it comes with serious consequences for an individual's health and well-being and society as a whole. Risk factors associated with illicit drug use involve a complex interaction of individual, biological and psychological variables within the social milieu and the individual's timeline. Conversely, factors associated with resilience can be identified and many of these have a self-efficacy basis. Interventions to increase resilience may be successful. Other interventions within a TRA framework and with underlying social marketing principles have been employed by the government to try to reduce substance misuse. Clinical interventions to prevent and/or treat illicit drug use are mainly based on cognitive and behavioural therapies or a combination of the two. Evaluation studies have generally supported the efficacy of such programmes in reducing illicit drug use.

Putting this into action

Consider Ricky's case:

- How would you assess his drug-taking behaviour?
- How would you assess all of his lifestyle behaviours?
- What type of drug user would you consider Ricky to be?
- What stage do you think Ricky is currently at?
- What do you need to do in order to move Ricky into the next stage?
- Develop an action plan for Ricky that focuses on reducing his drug taking, and prevents him relapsing.
- What sort of problems do you think Ricky will face whilst attempting to reduce his drug taking and how could you help him cope with these?

Summary points

- Substance misuse is now the generally accepted term for illicit drug use. There is no one generally accepted definition. Different definitions cover the purpose of drug taking, whether the behaviour is persistent and the consequences of the behaviour.
- Most cultures have laws associated with the misuse of drugs. What constitutes misuse and the seriousness of a particular transgression is culture bound and varies across time and between cultures.
- The WHO estimated that there were 185 million drug users worldwide in 2007. Ten per cent of the UK population report having taken illegal drugs in the preceding year and one-third of adults admit to having ever taken an illegal drug.
- Health consequences of illicit drug use include death and a variety of medical complaints dependent upon drug used. For example, cocaine use can result in heart attack, respiratory failure, stroke or seizures.

→

- Illicit drug use carries a significant financial cost. The HPA estimated that Class A drug users cost the UK economy £15.4 billion in 2003/2004.

- Multiple risk factors have been identified that increase the probability that an individual will engage in illicit drug use. Psychological risk factors include: anxiety, risk-taking and novelty-seeking tendencies. Socio-cultural factors include: drug availability, economic deprivation and peer group substance use. Demographic characteristics have also been implicated, and have genetic factors. There are complex interactions between these and other factors, and their influence varies over the lifespan.

- Protective variables such as parental responsibilities, career aspirations, lack of funds, fear of effects on health, negative personal experiences and self-efficacy have been identified as reducing the probability of illicit drug use.

- The gateway hypothesis proposes that use of 'softer' drugs (e.g. cannabis) is associated with the use of 'harder' drugs (e.g. cocaine, heroin) at a later time. There is evidence that the two are linked, although the causal mechanisms have not been identified.

- Social cognition models of illicit drug use suggest that drug use is determined by intention to perform the behaviour, which in turn is influenced by such things as attitudes, social norms, perceived control and self-efficacy. Studies have supported the predictive validity of social cognition models and interventions based upon them have been successful.

- Social marketing, using commercial marketing strategies to solve social and health problems, has been used in a number of other interventions, for example, FRANK. Studies investigating the effectiveness of such interventions have shown some support for a reduction in illicit drug use over the short term, but there is no evidence of a long-term effect as yet.

- There are a number of psychological interventions available to treat people with substance misuse problems. These include cognitive behavioural therapy, contingency management and motivational enhancement therapy. There is support for the effectiveness of these approaches.

Useful Web links

Alcoholics anonymous 0845 769 7555 http://www.alcoholics-anonymous.org.uk/

Talk to FRANK 0800 77 66 00 www.talktofrank.com/

Treatment guidelines for substance misuse http://www.dh.gov.uk/en/Publichealth/Healthimprovement/Drugmisuse/DH_085899

Department of Health – Live Well http://www.nhs.uk/LiveWell/Pages/Livewellhub.aspx

References

Andreasen, A.R. (2006). *Social Marketing in the 21st Centuary*. Thousand Oaks, CA: Sage.

American Psychiatric Association. (APA). (1994). *Diagnostic and Statistical Manual of Mental Disorders (DSM-IV)*. Washington, DC: American Psychiatric Association.

Bandura, A. (1977). *Social Learning Theory*. Englewood Cliffs, NJ: Prentice-Hall.

Bandura, A. (1986). *Social Foundations of Thought and Action: A Social Cognitive Theory.* Upper Saddle River, NJ: Prentice Hall.

Best, D., Gross, S., Manning, V., Gossop, M., Witton, J. and Strang, J. (2005). Cannabis use in adolescents: The impact of risk and protective factors and social functioning. *Drug and Alcohol Review,* 24, 483-488.

Boden, J.M., Fergusson, D.M. and Horwood, L.J. (2006). Illicit drug use and dependence in a New Zealand birth cohort. *Australian & New Zealand Journal of Psychiatry,* 40(2), 156-163.

Brown, R.L. and Rounds, L.A. (1995). Conjoint screening questionnaires for alcohol and drug abuse. *Wisconsin Medical Journal,* 94, 135-140.

Brown, R.L., Leonard, T., Saunders, L.A. and Papasouliotis, O.A. (2001). A two item conjoint screen for alcohol and other drug problems. *Journal of the American Board of Family Practice,* 14, 95-106.

Budney, A.J. and Higgins, S.T. (1998). A community *Reinforcement Plus Vouchers Approach: Treating Cocaine Addiction.* National Institute of Drug Abuse. NIH Pub. No. 98-4309. Washington, DC: US Government Printing Office.

Burke, B.L., Arkowitz, H. and Menchola, M. (2003). The efficacy of motivational interviewing: A meta-analysis of controlled clinical trials. *Journal of Consulting and Clinical Psychology,* 71, 843-861.

Carroll, K.M. and Onken, L.S. (2005). Behavioural therapies for drug abuse. *American Journal of Psychiatry,* 162, 1-9.

Condon, J. and Smith, N. (2003). *Prevalence of drug use: Key findings from the 2002/2003 British Crime Survey.* London: Home Office Findings 229.

Crowley, T.J. (1999). Research on contingency management treatment of drug dependence: Clinical implications and future directions. In S.T. Higgins and K. Silverman (eds) *Motivating Behaviour Change Among Illicit Drug Abusers* (pp. 345-370). Washington DC: American Psychological Association.

Deas, D. and Thomas, S.E. (2001). An overview of controlled studies of adolescent substance abuse treatment. *American Journal of Addiction,* 10(2), 178-189.

Dillon, L., Chivite-Matthews, N., Grewal, I., Brown, R., Webster, S., Weddell, E., Brown, G. and Smith, N. (2007). *Risk, protective factors and resilience to drug use: Identifying resilient young people and learning from their experiences.* Home Office online report. London: Home Office. Available at http://www.homeoffice.gov.uk/rds (accessed 27 November 2009).

Dunn, C., Deroo, L. and Rivara, F.P. (2001). The use of brief interventions adapted from motivational interviewing across behavioural domains: A systematic review. *Addiction,* 96, 1725-1742.

Epstein, J.A., Bang, H. and Botvin, G.J. (2007). Which psychosocial factors moderate or directly affect substance use among inner-city adolescents? *Addictive Behaviours,* 32, 700-713.

Ewing, J.A. (1984). Detecting alcoholism: The CAGE questionnaire. *Journal of the American Medical Association,* 252, 1905-1907.

Flynn, B.S., Worden, J.K., Secker-Walker, R.H., Pirie, P.L. Badger, G.J., Carpenter, J.H. and Geller, B.M. (1994). Mass-media and school interventions for cigarette smoking prevention: Effects 2 years after completion. *American Journal of Public Health,* 84, 1148-1150.

Frischer, M., Heatlie, H. and Hickman, M. (2004). *Estimating the prevalence of problematic and injecting drug use for Drug Action Team areas in England: A feasibility study using the Multiple Indicator Method.* Home Office online report 34/04. London: Home Office. Available at: http://www.homeoffice.gov.uk/rds/pdfs04/rdsolr3404.pdf (accessed 11 August 2008).

Gorsuch, R.L. (1980). Evaluating community based behavioral programs: Case example. In P. Schinke, Jr. (ed) *Community applications of behavioral methods: A sourcebook for social workers.* Hawthorne, NY: Aldine.

Irvin, J.E., Bowers, C.A., Dunn, M.E. and Wang, M.C. (1999). Efficacy of relapse prevention: A meta-analytic review. *Journal of Consulting and Clinical Psychology, 67,* 563–570.

Kandel, D.B. (2003). Does marijuana use cause use of other drugs? *Journal of the American Medical Association, 289,* 482–483.

Lee, N.K. and Rawson, R.A. (2008). A systematic review of cognitive and behavioural therapies for methamphetamine dependence. *Drug and Alcohol Review, 27,* 309–317.

Liddle, H.A., Dakof, G.A., Parker, K., Diamond, G.S., Barrett, K. and Tejeda, M. (2001). Multidimensional family therapy for adolescent drug abuse: Results of a randomized clinical trial. *The American Journal of Drug and Alcohol Abuse, 27,* 651–688.

Marlatt, G.A. and Gorden, G. (eds). (1985). *Relapse Prevention: Maintenance Strategies in Addictive Behavior Change.* New York: Guilford Press.

Marlatt, G.A. and Donovan, D.M. (eds). (2005). *Relapse Prevention: Maintenance Strategies in the Treatment of Addictive Behaviors* (2nd edn). New York: Guilford Press.

McGrath, Y.T., Sumnall, H.R., McVeigh, J. *et al.* (2006). *Review of Grey Literature on Drug Prevention among Young People.* London: NICE.

Mersy, D.J. (2003). Recognition of alcohol and substance abuse. *American Family Physician, 67,* 1529–1532.

Miller, W.R., Yahne, C.E. and Tonigan, J.S. (2003). Motivational interviewing in drug abuse services: a randomized trial. *Journal of Consulting and Clinical psychology, 71,* 754–763.

MTP Research Group. (2004). Brief treatments for cannabis dependence: Findings from a randomized multisite trial. *Journal of Consulting Clinical Psychology, 72,* 455–466.

National Institute for Health and Clinical Excellence (NICE). (2007). *Drug Misuse: Psychosocial Interventions.* London: NICE.

National Treatment Agency for Substance Misuse. (2005). *A National Survey of Inpatient Services in England.* London: The Stationery Office.

Nicholas, S., Kershaw, C. and Walker, K. (eds) (2008). *Crime in England and Wales 2006/7* (4th edn). London: Home Office.

NIDA (National Institute on Drug Abuse). (1997). *Preventing Drug Use among Children and Adolescents: A Research Based Guide.* National Institute of Health Publication No. 97-4212. Washington, DC: NIDA.

Office for National Statistics (ONS). (2000). Drug-related poisoning deaths: by selected type of drug, 1993 to 2000. *Social Trends,* 33. London: ONS.

Petraitis, J., Flay, B.R., and Miller, T.Q. (1995). Reviewing theories of adolescent substance use: Organising piece in the puzzle. *Psychological Bulletin, 117,* 67–86.

Prochaska, J.O., DiClemente, C.C. and Norcross, J.C. (1992). In search of how people change: Applications to addictive behaviours. *American Psychologist, 47,* 1102–1114.

Rohsenow, D.J., Monti, P.M., Martin, R.A., Michalec, E. and Abrams, D.B. (2000). Brief coping skills treatment for cocaine abuse: 12-month substance use outcomes. *Journal Consulting Clinical Psychology,* 68, 515–520.

Sareen, J., Chartier, M., Paulus, M.P. and Stein, M.B. (2006). Illicit drug use and anxiety disorders: Findings from two community surveys. *Psychiatry Research,* 122(1), 11–17.

Spooner, C. (1999). Causes and correlates of adolescent drug abuse and implications for treatment. *Drug & Alcohol Review,* 18(4), 453–475.

Stephens, R.S., Roffman, R.A. and Curtain, L. (2000). Comparison of extended versus brief treatments for marijuana use. *Journal of Consulting and clinical Psychology,* 68, 898–908.

Stitzer, M.L., Iguchi, M.Y. and Felch, L.J. (1992). Contingent takehome incentive: Effects on drug use of methadone maintenance patients. *Journal of Consulting and Clinical Psychology,* 60, 927–934.

Sumnall, H.R. and Bellis, M.A. (2007). Can health campaigns make people ill? The iatrogenic potential of population-based cannabis prevention. *Journal of Epidemiology and Community Health,* 61, 930–931.

Velleman, R., Mistral, W. and Sanderling, L. (1999). Parents and drugs prevention. In *Evaluating Effectiveness: Drugs Prevention Research Conference Paper 20.* London: Home Office, DPI.

Velleman, R.D.B., Templeton, L.J. and Copello, A.G. (2005). The role of the family in preventing and intervening with substance use and misuse: A comprehensive review of family interventions, with a focus on young people. *Drug & Alcohol Review,* 24(2), 93–109.

WHO. (2007a). International Classification of Diseases (10th rev.). Available at: http://www.who.int/classifications/apps/icd/icd10online/ (accessed 23 November 2009).

WHO. (2007b). Global burden of substance abuse. Available at: http://www.who.int/substance_abuse/facts/global_burden/en/index.html (accessed 23 November 2009).

Wiebe, G.D. (1951–1952). Merchandising commodities and citizenship on television. *Public Opinion Quarterly,* 15, 679–91.

Chapter 9
Conclusion

LEARNING OBJECTIVES

At the end of this chapter you will:

- Appreciate the differences between an interventionist and a libertarian approach to health promotion
- Understand the current public health policy
- Recognise the practitioner role in behavioural change
- Recognise the difficulties faced by individuals attempting to change
- Have considered future directions for health promotion

Sex, food, drink and smoking: either an enjoyable night out or a potential time bomb, depending on your perspective. This book has addressed these behaviours (and drugs and lack of exercise) from a psychological perspective – exploring how psychology can explain such behaviours and how it can be used to modify unsafe practices. This does not mean that we, or other promoters of healthy lifestyle, should be labelled as kill-joys or party poopers. It just means that we advocate changing lifestyle for the better, to improve health and to promote life expectancy: you cannot enjoy yourself if you are dead from coronary heart disease, lung cancer or some other 'lifestyle disease'.

This concluding chapter will explore the role of psychological interventions within a political and social context. Although the techniques, research and evidence we have presented within this book will be of use to the individual healthcare professional, it is important that the policy framework is recognised. Whilst it is beyond the scope of this text to explore all of these elements and there are other books that take a more socio-political perspective on lifestyle (e.g. Thirlaway and Upton, 2009), it is essential that the healthcare professional appreciates the context in which they work. Consequently, this chapter will outline the lifestyle policy in the UK since the 1990s and how this impacts on the ethics of intervention and individual practice.

Health professionals promoting evidence-based strategies (and we have tried to concentrate on these research or evidence-based methods) for lifestyle change face criticism and competition from many sources, many of whom base their critiques and alternative solutions on personal experience. For example, Janet Street-Porter in the *Independent on Sunday* (2008a) claimed that 'Obesity is a result of wilful self-abuse' rather than offering any coherent psychological explanation. Similarly, as we pointed out at the outset of this text, Rod Liddle in the *Sunday Times* suggested that: 'Most obesity is a consequence of stupidity and indolence and not of some genetic affliction. It is a lifestyle choice which people would be less inclined to adopt if they knew we all hated them for it' (Liddle, 2008).

Such columnists are often opposed to any strategy that limits personal choice and have accused the government of building a 'nanny state'. However, Janet Street-Porter had changed her mind a month later and was proposing rationing of sugar, chocolate, fats and salt (Street-Porter, 2008b). Janet-Street Porter has also thrown her oar into the debate about how to curb drinking. She confidently stated, in direct contradiction to the actual research evidence (Room 2004), that: 'there is absolutely no evidence that making drink more expensive will have any effect on the number of people getting slaughtered night after night' (Street-Porter, 2008c). It is the job of columnists like Janet Street-Porter and Rod Liddle to write controversial text, so we can take some of their comments with a pinch of salt (although no more than 6 g per day). Of course, it is encouraging that lifestyle diseases and lifestyle behaviours are finally getting media coverage and that the health problems that arise from unsafe sex, binge drinking and so on are front-page news. It was not long ago that Harrabin *et al.* (2003) were voicing concern at the media's lack of interest in lifestyle diseases. What is concerning, however, is that everybody now sees themselves as an expert on lifestyle, and alongside the columnists creating controversy are a plethora of lay persons offering health and lifestyle advice that ranges from the ill-advised to the positively dangerous. Consequently, this text sets out to offer fundamentally sensible advice based on psychological principles supported by consistent and high-quality research.

Of course, the healthcare professional does not operate within a vacuum – and there is a need for the healthcare professional to appreciate the socio-economic and policy environment in which their practice occurs. Prevention of lifestyle diseases through promoting healthy lifestyle choices has been a central tenet of health policy in the UK since 1999 (Department of Health, 1999). The government faces two interrelated challenges. Firstly, they need to change the established lifestyle habits of the current generation of adults, and secondly, they need to prevent the next generation of adults establishing similar or worse lifestyle habits. Lifestyle policy in the UK addresses these two issues, firstly by attempting to modify cultural norms. For example, in an attempt to promote sensible drinking the policy has been to shape the environment – to change the cultural norms to one of sensible and safe drinking rather than one characterised by binge drinking (HM Government, 2007). However, what has to be recognised is that this will be a long and generational process: 'cultures exist where being active or eating 'healthy' foods are not top priorities' (Jones *et al.*, 2007, p. 38). Furthermore, it is important to appreciate that culture is difficult to change, especially if people do not have the resources to change: 'the behaviour of these individuals may be the most difficult to modify due to both the difficulties in reaching them and overcoming their norms' (Jones *et al.*, 2007, p. 38) irrespective of the amount of facilities and support available to them. As Alan Johnson (the UK's Health Secretary) stated: 'The causes of poor health are not so much about the choices people make, *but the choices they are able to make*' (Speech by Alan Johnson, 19 March 2009).

Changing cultural norms could both establish healthy lifestyle habits from the outset and make it easier for individuals to change established unhealthy lifestyles, and there would no longer be a need for this book. Lifestyle policy clearly aims to direct cultural trends (HM Government, 2007: Department of Health, 1999; Jones *et al.*, 2007) but is itself a product of our history and culture. For instance, there is no clear scientific rationale for a drug like cannabis to be illegal whilst a drug like alcohol is not. Alcohol is an integral part of our history and culture and banning it in Britain has never been considered a viable response to the problems that arise from drinking. The opening statement of 'Safe. Sensible. Social' (HM Government, 2007) makes it clear that alcohol is seen as a primarily positive aspect of society despite the severe behavioural and health consequences. The same document goes on to report that 'Alcohol can play an important and positive role in British culture' (HM Government, 2007).

A population-level approach to public health interventions has always been assumed to be the most cost-effective and efficient way to produce behavioural change. It is cheaper and can get the message to a greater number of individuals than the clinical measures ever can, and it will result (hopefully) in the development of cultural changes. The most significant population-level smoking intervention in recent years has been legislation to restrict smoking in public places. Since March 2006 in Scotland, April 2007 in Northern Ireland and Wales, and July 2007 in England, all public places and workplaces have been smoke free. The introduction of this change was not particularly controversial – the proportion of the population supporting such a change was high. Of course, commentators such as Rod Liddle have argued strongly against the ban. For example, when commenting on the smoking ban introduced by Sir Liam Donaldson, the Chief Medical Officer: 'Sir Liam is the chap who believes today's unjust and draconian smoking ban is "only a start" and wishes to pursue smokers into the family home. Despite evidence to the contrary, Donaldson believes passive smoking kills millions of people; but then his career has been built upon scaring people' (Liddle, 2007). However, it appears that this 'draconian ban' has already reduced the number of heart attacks in the UK. It may be draconian but it is clearly effective, and more effective than decades of anti-smoking promotion activities (Pell and Haw, 2009).

An interesting perspective and debate was raised by the Nuffield Council on Bioethics (2007) who argued that public health policies should be about enforcement. They proposed an 'intervention ladder' as a useful way of conceptualising public health interventions and their impact on an individual's choice (see Table 9.1). In the case of smoking, how does this fit into the ladder? It can be seen that currently the government 'guides by disincentives' and 'restricts choice' to a certain extent. The ban on smoking in public places is significant as it is the first legislative attempt to alter lifestyle choices made by governments for many years. However, surely it can be argued that the government should totally eliminate choice, i.e. we should ban smoking. On the one hand, smoking is a behaviour which is avoidable – society and civilisation would not suffer considerably if it was banned across the country. Certainly, the Nuffield Council on Bioethics (2007) would argue that this would be important and that enforcement should be used and this curtailment of individual freedom would be ethically justified. Their argument concerns proportionality – can the enforcement benefits outweigh the interference in people's lives? Smoking is a dangerous lifestyle behaviour that has its roots in social, physiological and psychological elements. Its dangers are obvious to most and it can kill not only the individual but the innocent bystander. Is this sufficient to 'eliminate choice' (to use the phrasing of the Nuffield Council, aka 'ban', 'coerce' or 'outlaw')? Obviously, libertarians would argue that smoking is a right of the individual and if individuals want to choose this behaviour then this is their right. Consequently, it is up to health promoters, health psychologists and healthcare professionals to promote smoking cessation and not to severely curtail our freedoms. An editorial in the London Times (13 November 2007) argues that 'John Stuart Mill held that the only justification for state coercion was to prevent harm, or "evil", being done to others. It is a stretch to say that . . . smoking at home meets this definition.'

Laws that eliminate or restrict lifestyle choices are generally in place to protect others from harm, not the individuals themselves. Consequently, people can no longer smoke in a public place in order to protect others, and driving under the influence of alcohol is illegal. Critics of such interventionist policies (including Janet Street-Porter, Dominic Lawson and Rod Liddle) have argued that such measures are 'nanny state-ist' (Jochelson, 2006) and an unnecessary intrusion into people's personal lives. The current government, and the official opposition, distance themselves from such interventionist attitudes, although the current health secretary did teasingly ask 'is it too great a leap to assume that what works today for smoking will also work for obesity, or for that matter alcohol?' (Johnson, 2009). However, this debate about the limits to state freedom and public health is not new. Libertarians have long argued that minimal state intervention is the way to protect individual freedom. For example, a commentator suggested that the original Public Health Act of 1848 was 'paternalistic' and 'despotic' and 'a little dirt and freedom' was 'more desirable than no dirt at all and slavery' (Porter, 1999).

From the other end of the intervention ladder (Table 9.1) the government remains committed to a policy of guiding choice, despite the irrefutable evidence across all lifestyle behaviours that educational and risk communication messages do not have any significant effect on lifestyle choices (Floyd et al., 2000; Milne et al., 2000; Blue, 2007; Ruiter, 2004; Taubman Ben-Ari and Findler, 2005). Attempts to develop a culture of sensible drinking have been a dismal failure and young women are actually drinking more than ever. However, cultural norms can be modified; drink-driving is no longer considered an acceptable behaviour and drink-related road accidents have been reduced. Smoking in public places is no longer acceptable and the move to this position was not nearly as contentious as was feared (ONS, 2005). However, all these cultural shifts have been supported by clear legislation; it is unlikely that health promotion alone will change lifestyle culture.

Table 9.1 The intervention ladder

Level	Description	Example
Eliminate choice	Introduce laws that entirely eliminate choice	Compulsory isolation of those with an infectious disorder
Restrict choice	Introduce laws that restrict the options available to people	Remove unhealthy foods from shops
Guide through disincentives	Introduce financial or other disincentives to influence behaviour	Increase taxes on cigarettes
Guide through incentives	Introduce financial or other incentives to influence people's behaviour	Tax breaks for bicycle purchases
Guide choices	Changing the default policy	Change the standard side dish from chips to salad
Enable choice	Help individuals to change their behaviour	Free stop-smoking programmes
Provide information	Inform and educate public	Encourage people to eat five portions of fruit/veg a day
Do nothing	Or monitor situation	

Source: Nuffield Council on Bioethics (2007)

In the context of this social and policy background, the healthcare practitioner has to promote healthy behaviour and behaviour change. The government has set many targets around reducing the incidence of lifestyle diseases and their main strategy to achieve these goals is to increase healthy and decrease unhealthy lifestyle choices. However, although the healthcare professional has a fundamental role, they are not the only one that has a responsibility for improving health and behavioural choices. For example, in the alcohol policy document 'Safe. Sensible. Social' (HM Government, 2007), virtually all public servants - the police, local authorities, the NHS, schools, voluntary organisations - are tasked with delivering the government's strategy. Furthermore, the government also identifies the alcohol industry and the wider business industry, the media and local communities as having a role to play in delivering their strategy. However, who is to deliver the behavioural change component of this strategy, which receives scant attention in the document but has the clearest evidence-base as to its efficacy, is not addressed (Moyer et al., 2002; Mulvihill et al., 2005; Poikolainen, 1999; Williams et al., 2007). Similarly, various public servants and businesses are involved in the promotion of healthy eating and physical activity but the central question of who should deliver the essential behavioural change component of the strategy remains unclear.

Of course, the principal candidates for the delivery of behavioural change interventions are primary care practitioners: general practitioners, practice nurses, health visitors and other associated healthcare professionals (Ashenden et al., 1997). Primary care has been central in the delivery of individual lifestyle advice for some time, and there is conflicting evidence about whether merely advising patients to change their lifestyle can lead to lifestyle change (Ashenden et al., 1997; Moyer et al., 2002). However, it is clear that a psychologically based intervention is more likely to be successful (Moyer et al., 2002; Biddle et al., 1997). To give healthcare professionals the best chance of delivering psychologically based lifestyle interventions they will need more than a copy of this book. Here we simply introduce the key concepts and ideas. Healthcare professionals will need training and resources if they are to deliver the changes in behaviour that governments are looking for.

In England, a new initiative to promote lifestyle change has been launched: health trainers with a specific remit of promoting healthy lifestyles in the community. These health trainers are being taught the key psychological techniques identified in this text to enable them to support individuals in their community to adopt healthy lifestyle habits. Whilst the establishment of psychologically trained 'health trainers' is an important step forward in improving the health of society, many other health professionals will still need to address lifestyle change with their patients.

In order to deliver effective preventative lifestyle interventions, health practitioners will need a range of resources and skills. Firstly, they will need to be able to measure current lifestyle behaviours quickly and reliably and to recognise individuals who have severe problems that need referral to a specialist. Within each of the chapters we have presented information on how to assess, and there may be many such techniques. Importantly, the individual healthcare professional needs to be able to recognise the limits of their expertise and refer on as appropriate. So, for example, they need to be able to recognise the difference between substance use, misuse and addiction and refer on for specialist help as appropriate.

Health professionals who wish to enable the patients they work with to change their lifestyle first and foremost need to recognise that simply providing people with information about the risks of unhealthy lifestyles will not result in lifestyle change. If health professionals wish to encourage lifestyle change they should be looking to increase self-motivation, increase self-regulatory skills, set achievable goals and increase self-efficacy in their clients. Although reading this text has been a start, it is not a finishing point: there are additional seminars, courses and resources available that healthcare professionals need to make use of.

We are at a turning point in health promotion. The ineffectiveness of the previous decades of educational interventions is irrefutable and policy makers and health professionals are both starting to recognise the importance of psychological processes in lifestyle change (Thirlaway and Upton, 2009). Fortunately, psychology is a discipline with a strong record of high-quality research and we are already in a position to provide evidence-based advice about appropriate psychological interventions. Lifestyle behaviours are extremely varied but nevertheless the same psychological constructs are relevant to promoting change in them all. The potential opportunity to develop training and protocols for interventions that can be applied across all lifestyle behaviours should not be ignored.

Conclusion

This final chapter has attempted to pull together the material presented throughout this text within a social and policy context. It is important that the healthcare professional recognises the key role of public policy in the promotion of healthy lifestyle and their individual practice. The chapter stresses the tension between the libertarian perspective currently predominant in our society and the evidence that a more interventionist approach to public health policy can have a significant impact on health and well-being.

Motivation and self-efficacy have been established as key cognitive factors in successful lifestyle change. For now, the healthcare professional needs to maximise intervention-based knowledge and to develop and enhance self-efficacy as a key route for lifestyle change. However, we need to explore further the role of non-cognitive factors such as habitual responses and enjoyment in the establishment of lifestyle choices. We need to develop research protocols, evidence-based interventions and strategies that can extend our under-standing and implementation of successful lifestyle change. People do not usually make ini-tial lifestyle choices based on future health implications and by the time they wish to protect their health they need to overcome well-established bad habits. Ultimately we hope that the material in this text becomes redundant and the focus alters from changing unhealthy behaviours to maintaining healthy ones.

Summary points

- Everyone is an expert on lifestyle change and often advice is based on personal experience of change rather than research evidence.
- There is a tension between libertarian and interventionist approaches to public health.
- Restricting lifestyle choices through legislation can play an important role in changing cultural norms and individual behaviour and in improving long-term health.
- Healthcare professionals have a key role in promoting behaviour change.
- A psychological approach to lifestyle change can play a central role in the development of a healthy society.

References

Ashenden, R., Silagy, C. and Weller, D. (1997). A systematic review of the effectiveness of pro-moting lifestyle change in general practice. *Family Practice*, 14, 160-174.

A Sugared Pill: The Nuffield Council tries, but fails, to justify the nanny state (2007, 13 November). *London Times*. Available at: http://www.timesonline.co.uk/tol/comment/leading_article/article2859367.ece (accessed 23 September 2009).

Biddle, S., Edmunds, L., Bowler, I. and Killoran, A. (1997). Physical activity promotion through primary health care in England. *British Journal of General Practice*, 47 (419), 367-369.

Blue, C.L. (2007). Does the theory of planned behaviour identify diabetes-related cognitions for intention to be physically active and eat a healthy diet? *Public Health Nursing*, 24(2), 141-150.

Department of Health (DoH). (1999). *Saving Lives: Our Healthier Nation*. London: The Stationery Office.

Floyd, D.L., Prentice-Dunn, S. and Rogers, R.W. (2000). A meta-analysis of protection motiva-tion theory. *Journal of Applied Social Psychology*, 30, 407-429.

Harrabin, R., Coote, A. and Allen, J. (2003). *Health in the News: Risk, Reporting and Media Influence*. London: King's Fund.

HM Government. (2007). *Safe, Sensible, Social. The Next Steps in the National Alcohol Strategy*. London: Department of Health and The Home Office.

Jochelson, K. (2006). Nanny or steward? The role of government in public health. *Public Health*, 120, 1149-1155.

Johnston, A. (2009). 'Nanny state, Nudge State or No state?' Royal Society of Arts, London, 19 March.

Jones, A., Bentham, G., Foster, C., Hillsdon, M. and Panter, J. (2007). *Tackling Obesities: Future Choices – Obesogenic Environments – Evidence Review*. London: Foresight.

Liddle, R. (2007). So that's his real NHS priority – a £2 billion stealth cut in England. *Sunday Times*, 1 July.

Liddle, R. (2008). Laugh at lard butts – but just remember Fatty Fritz lives longer. *Sunday Times*, 27 January.

Milne, S., Sheeran, P. and Orbell, S. (2000). Prediction and intervention in health-related behaviour: A meta review of protection motivation theory. *Journal of Applied Social Psychology*, 30, 106-143.

Moyer, A., Finney, J.W., Swearingen, E. and Vergun, P. (2002). Brief interventions for alcohol problems: A meta-analytic review of controlled investigations in treatment seeking and non-treatment seeking populations. *Addiction*, 97, 279-292.

Mulvihill, C., Taylor, L., Waller, S., Naidoo, B. and Thom, B. (2005). *Prevention and Reduction of Alcohol Misuse: Evidence Briefing*, 2nd edn. London: Health Development Agency.

Nuffield Council on Bioethics. (2007). *Public Health Ethical Issues*. London: Nuffield Council. www.nuffieldbioethics.org

Office for National Statistics (ONS). (2005). *Smoking-related Behaviour and Attitudes, 2005*. London: HMSO.

Pell, J.P. and Haw, S. (2009). The triumph of national smoke free legislation. *Heart,* 95, 1377-1380.

Poikolainen, K. (1999). Effectiveness of brief interventions to reduce alcohol intake in primary care populations: A meta analysis. *Preventative Medicine,* 28, 503-509.

Porter, D. (1999). *Health, Civilisation and the State. A History of Public Health from Ancient to Modern Times.* London: Routledge.

Room, R. (2004). Disabling the public interest: Alcohol strategies and policies for England. *Addiction,* 99, 1083-1089.

Ruiter, R.A.C. (2004). *Effecten van angstaanjagende tv-spotjes [Effects of fear-arousing TV commercials]. Final report.* Maastricht, Netherlands: Maastricht University, Department of Experimental Psychology.

Street-Porter, J. (2008a). Let the adult fatties eat themselves to death. The kids we can save. *Independent on Sunday,* 27 January.

Street-Porter, J. (2008b). A return to the ration book is the answer to obesity. *Independent on Sunday,* 24 February.

Street-Porter, J. (2008c). Don't blame it on the young, we're a nation of boozers. *Independent on Sunday,* 24 February.

Taubman Ben-Ari, O. and Findler, L. (2005). Proximal and distal effects of mortality salience on willingness to engage in health promoting behavior along the life span. *Psychology & Health,* 20, 303-318.

Thirlaway, K. and Upton, D. (2009). *The Psychology of Lifestyle: Promoting Healthy Behaviour.* London: Routledge.

Williams, E.C., Horton, N.J., Samet, J.H. and Saitz, R. (2007). Do brief measures of readiness to change predict alcohol consumption and consequences in primary care patients with unhealthy alcohol use? *Alcoholism: Clinical and Experimental Research,* 31, 428-435.

Index